THE ULTIMATE TOXIC MOLD RECOVERY GUIDE
TAKE BACK YOUR HOME, HEALTH & LIFE

BRIDGIT DANNER, LAC, FDNP

CONTENTS

Foreword — xi
Introduction: My Mold Story — xiii

Part I
DISCOVER

1. WHAT IS TOXIC MOLD? — 3
   - In This Chapter — 3
   - Introduction — 3
   - What Is Toxic Mold? — 4
   - The Aspects of Mold That Make You Sick — 6
   - Toxic Mold Over Time — 8
   - Where Toxic Mold Is Found — 10
   - What Encourages Mold Growth — 11
   - Summary — 16

2. HOW TO ASSESS YOUR HOME & BODY FOR TOXIC MOLD — 19
   - In This Chapter — 19
   - How to Assess Your Home & Body — 20
   - What to Test — 38
   - Summary — 41

3. HOW CAN TOXIC MOLD AFFECT YOUR HEALTH — 43
   - In This Chapter — 43
   - Introduction — 43
   - Mold Terminology — 44
   - Mold & Your Health History — 45
   - Mold & Your Genetics — 46
   - The Trouble with Mycotoxins — 48
   - Mold & Your Body Systems — 49
   - Toxic Mold & Your Hormones — 50
   - Summary — 61

4. NEXT STEPS & FINDING SUPPORT	65
In This Chapter	65
Introduction	65
Next Steps	66
Chunking it Down	67
Prioritizing	68
Deciding Factors	71
Finding Grace in the Chaos	71
Resource Survey	72
Sharing & Asking for Help	75
Summary	78

Part II
DO

5. WHAT TO DO ABOUT YOUR HOME & BELONGINGS	83
In This Chapter	83
Introduction	83
Moving 101	85
Shopping	100
Insurance	102
Legal Rights	103
Summary	104
6. PREPARING FOR A SAFE & SMOOTH BODY DETOX	107
In This Chapter	107
Introduction	107
What's the Best Order of Detox?	108
Open Your Detox Pathways	110
Special Conditions	118
Working with Children	119
Supplements	120
Have a Physician & Work with Experts	121
Summary	122

7. STEP 1: MASTER THE FOUNDATIONS OF GOOD HEALTH — 125
   - In This Chapter — 125
   - Introduction — 125
   - Nature Time — 126
   - Toxin Avoidance — 128
   - Movement — 128
   - Rest & Self-Care — 131
   - Sleep Well — 132
   - Hydration — 132
   - Alignment to Your Values and Mission — 134
   - Quality Relationships — 136
   - Eat a MATH Diet — 138
   - Essential Supplementation — 142
   - Summary — 145

8. MORE ON DIET — 147
   - In This Chapter — 147
   - Introduction — 147
   - How to Eat — 150
   - Special Dietary Considerations — 152
   - 15 Foods that Grow Mold Easily — 153
   - How to Avoid Mold in Foods — 153
   - Food Dos and Don'ts — 163
   - Summary — 165

9. STEP 2: ESTABLISH YOUR DETOX ROUTINE — 167
   - In This Chapter: — 167
   - Introduction — 167
   - Why & How to Detox — 168
   - My Top Supplements — 169
   - My Top Techniques — 182
   - Summary — 192

10. MORE DETOX TECHNIQUES — 193
    - In This Chapter — 193
    - Introduction — 193
    - Detox Techniques A-Z — 194
    - Summary: — 213

11. **STEP 3: TARGETED SYMPTOM/SYSTEM REPAIR** — 215
    - In This Chapter — 215
    - Introduction — 215
    - Fatigue — 216
    - Cell Danger Response (CDR) — 218
    - Brain Fog — 219
    - Pain / Headaches — 222
    - Digestive Complaints — 224
    - Weight Gain/Food Cravings/Energy Fluctuations — 229
    - Immune/Respiratory Issues — 232
    - Mental Health Issues — 235
    - Chemical Sensitivities — 237
    - Poor Sleep — 240
    - Hormonal Imbalance — 242
    - Conclusion — 244

12. **MORE ABOUT LAB OPTIONS** — 247
    - In This Chapter — 247
    - Introduction — 247
    - Blood Tests — 248
    - Urine Tests — 250
    - Hair Testing — 253
    - Stool Tests — 254
    - Scans — 255

Part III
DEVELOP

13. **AVOID ALL TOXINS** — 261
    - In This Chapter — 261
    - Introduction — 261
    - Sources of Toxins — 263
    - Inspecting Your Home for Toxins — 270
    - Conclusion — 276

14. **STAGE OF HEALING** — 279
    - In This Chapter — 279
    - Introduction — 279
    - Stages of Healing — 280

Health is Never Static	281
Routine vs. Variety	282
Conclusions	284
15. CREATING A NEW LIFE YOU LOVE	287
In This Chapter	287
Introduction	287
Reflect on Your Life	288
Out With the Old, In With the New	296
Your Turn	301
Acknowledgments	303
About the Author	307

This book is not intended to replace your relationship with your physician. Please seek guidance before beginning this or any new medical program.

Copyright © 2022 by Bridgit Danner, LAc, FDN-P

All rights reserved. No part of this book may be reproduced or used in any manner without written permission of the copyright owner except for the use of quotations in a book review.

First paperback edition April 2022

Book design by Melissa Cardenas

ISBN 978-0-578-35556-6

www.bridgitdanner.com

To my parents, who have stood by me through my wildest dreams and darkest hours.

FOREWORD

I've known Bridgit Danner for several years. When I met her she still owned an integrative wellness center and was pursuing another big passion, her online business in women's health. I was in the same field, and we quickly bonded over our desire to really serve women.

She was always eager to learn anything new about health and practiced what she preached.

I don't think I realized how much she was struggling with her health until I heard she had moved out of her house, too affected by toxic mold to live there anymore.

Even still, she was getting work done and taking care of her family. I watched her bounce around from state to state and home to home, and still she didn't give up on her business - teaching women about hormones and publishing books on fertility.

Like me, Bridgit is a lil' type A personality with a big drive! But behind that drive to work was also a drive to serve. She didn't

FOREWORD

want to give up on her dreams or the women she wanted to reach.

It took Bridgit a long time to realize that mold was behind her ongoing hormonal problems. And it would be a major pivot for her business to change from teaching hormones to teaching mold.

But once she started to get better, I saw her dedication to teaching detoxification in a big way so that other men and women could know that their own hormonal issues - along with brain fog, fatigue and more - might be due to toxic mold.

I am so proud to see how far she's come and I know how hard she struggled as she focused on healing herself and her family from the effects of toxic mold. Now she is using her experience and expertise to help many other families reclaim their health and lives too after toxic mold exposure. This book is a culmination of everything that she has researched and applied to thousands of people just like you.

She's created a fabulous, comprehensive resource for anyone struggling with a moldy home or body. I hope it will help you struggle a lot less, and feel supported along the way by all the care she has for you.

Dr. Mariza Synder
Best-selling author of *The Essential Oils Hormone Solution: Reclaim Your Energy and Focus and Lose Weight Naturally*

INTRODUCTION: MY MOLD STORY

It's hard to keep any mold story short and sweet, but I wanted to share a timeline of my experience straight away, and I promise to share some of my happy discoveries and wins as we get into the book!

2006 - The Start of It All

This year was a year of beautiful beginnings, but also the year I unwittingly moved into a moldy home.

I got engaged and moved in with my future husband. His home happened to be a 100-year old hodge-podge of renovations and additions in the rainy city of Portland, Oregon.

I was also starting my own full-fledged integrative clinic, so I was busy and stressed.

I was anxious to start a family because I was 33 and, at the time, I thought that was old!

So I piled wedding planning, family planning, and opening a business into one year, and it was a horrible idea in retrospect.

I wasn't sleeping well but I got pregnant easily.

2007 - Baby Boy & Baby Symptoms

I had a rough pregnancy but worked hard throughout to support my new business. I was super stressed and occasionally puking in the alley behind my clinic.

My back hurt all the time and my diet was not great - I fueled my energy needs with an occasional bag of powdered doughnuts. All my symptoms were attributed to a normal pregnancy during my doctors' visits.

My son was born healthy and beautiful and it was an exciting time.

2008 - The Sh*t Hits the Fan

I'd say this was the year that things got bad. Stress turned into anxiety. A happy marriage turned into loneliness and anger. My immune system was struggling. I got pink eye. And my back still hurt all the time.

I got off hormonal birth control in the hopes that it would calm my moods. I got a life coach and tried to find balance. I started eating better and got off gluten and dairy, at least mostly.

2009-2014 - Treading Water

These years were just more of the same. I was working very hard, raising a young child, running a household mostly on my own, and trying my best to feel better in my body.

Sometimes I felt better (usually in the summer), but often I still felt crappy. I got a cold or flu about every 2 weeks. My periods were irregular. I had chronic pain and insomnia. My digestion was good because I ate really carefully, but I was very rigid with my family about our diet.

I was becoming a skilled acupuncturist, and studying functional medicine and nutrition on the side, trying to resolve my own symptoms.

2015 - The Tipping Point

The day after Thanksgiving in 2015 was a severe tipping point for my health.

I got strep throat that required antibiotics, my first dose in 20 years. And I didn't recover after that. I was exhausted. I did a detox program - didn't help. I got IV vitamin therapy - didn't help.

I was working from home on my online business. **I was home nearly all the time during a very rainy fall in Portland, Oregon that caused visible leaking in our already musty basement.**

I was getting IV therapy at our local naturopathic school, and I asked them for some advanced testing. I was literally doing everything I could for my health and I was BONE TIRED.

They ran some tests for autoimmunity but the most critical thing they asked me was if anything had changed in my home. This was my first conversation about possible mold in my home.

Some positive test results I received dovetailed with toxic mold illness. These were:

- Parasites
- Candida
- Leaky gut
- Food sensitivities
- Low sex hormone production
- Low adrenal hormone production

- Epstein-Barr virus positive
- Low thyroid hormone levels
- Hashimoto's thyroiditis
- Low white blood cell count
- Low ferritin

You might be thinking, *Man, that's an awful lot of testing!* I found out I had mold soon after completing my Functional Diagnostic Nutrition training course, so I got a lot of tests run as a student, and then got more during this health low point.

2016 - The Reveal & Move #1

In our home, we used a local mold inspector as a starting point, and then later ran a mycotoxin test for dust. We had a great inspector, and I'm very thankful we made that first step.

We received an inspection report that was positive for toxic mold and water damage, and moved forward with a first round of remediation. **We made several mistakes in the process of remediation, so pay close attention to the upcoming chapters if you'll be remediating.**

As things got worse, my energy was even lower and my brain was functioning poorly, and I resisted moving out both due to the inconvenience and my sheer exhaustion. **I lost things, had a horrible short-term memory, and was so tired that I had suicidal thoughts - my body was begging for a relief for the fatigue.**

We did move into free, temporary housing (a house my parents had recently bought to move closer to us), which was a blessing for our health but a major pain for commuting. My husband was also experiencing fatigue and some other symptoms; luckily our son had no overt symptoms.

We made the error of moving more of our items into their home than we should have. We transported these items in our cars. We ended up ruining both cars *and* the new home environment with the mycotoxin transfer.

We stayed in this temporary home for about 4-6 months while our home had further repairs, including all new siding, some new structural beams and flooring, new carpet and a new deck.

We tossed, sold or stored away everything we owned and got the house ready to sell. The technical work we hired out, but the non-technical work we did ourselves, except for hiring a cleaning team for a floor-to-ceiling wipe down.

This was all incredibly expensive. I'm not even sure how we afforded it, but we knew once the house sold, we'd get the money back. We were lucky to sell in a hot sellers' market.

We had another mold inspection; it passed and we sold the home in the summer of 2016.

Because our mold was all due to building errors (by the previous owner and not identified in the buying process) and developed over time, nothing was covered by insurance.

I was self-employed and had no insurance to take a leave from work. My then-husband eventually got a paid medical leave for two months, and we went on a two-month trip to Arizona, Colorado, California and Nevada to dry out, heal and re-evaluate. I worked remotely the best I could.

The trip was really great for our family and I recommend doing something similar if you can.

When we returned to Portland two months later, we struggled to find a home we felt safe about. We did find a lovely place, although we could not use the ground-level office due to mold (long story).

That winter in Portland was especially wet and snowy. My then-husband was reacting to a moldy lab at his workplace, which his employers did not take seriously. My health got worse again in this climate, and my stress was through the roof with my return to clinic work, an online business, and a marriage on the rocks.

We decided to leave Oregon for Arizona although we waited for the school year to end first. Before leaving, we had to sort through stored belongings, which re-exposed us to mold.

2017 - Move #2

I worked hard to find a buyer for my Portland clinic and eventually I found an amazing woman who was ready to start a new life on the West coast.

Although there *is* indoor mold in Arizona, it's much less common due to the dry climate. We felt good about the house we moved into, and we got new non-toxic, full-house flooring right away which eliminated leftover dust and chemicals.

After settling in, I realized I was still sick. Not as sick as before, but up and down sick. I remember I was still doing nasal rinses daily to deal with post-nasal drip. It had been nearly two years since we discovered mold, so this was disappointing. I think I had unconsciously thought I'd be in perfect health after moving.

I still had some mold in my body at this point (I tested in the Spring of 2018), but I think I mostly was dealing with all the other issues that had developed. I treated myself for parasites and Epstein Barr virus. I bought my first sauna.

2018 & 2019 - A Slow Climb Back to Health

These years I slowly got better and better. I'd say mental fatigue from working was my biggest challenge. I also had frequent sore throats and swollen glands in my neck which I thought was due to Epstein Barr virus, but then later suspected was due to candida. I developed asthma.

In 2019 my husband moved out and filed for divorce. The stress of it all greatly contributed to my anxiety, poor sleep and poor appetite.

2020 - COVID & Move #3

When COVID hit in 2020, it seemed like child's play compared to going through a divorce. Despite everything going on, I'd say my health was better than ever this year.

I solved my sore throats with mouth taping and I had the best wintertime immunity than I'd had in many years.

I moved into my own home in 2020, which was exciting but also pretty ungrounding and I hit my head and got a bad concussion. It was exacerbated due to pre-existing neck tension, and I eventually recovered.

2021 - WTF Does This Ever End ?*!

Ok I am just joking with this title, but if you look back on your recent years you may feel the same way! **Life is a series of upheavals, meaningful milestones and lots of little moments in between.**

I certainly haven't mastered being in the moment and in gratitude all the time, but I have gotten better at it. I meditate daily with the Insight Timer app. I have coaches and counselors and really good friends. I have a great family and work team.

When something doesn't feel right, I might need a new perspective or a tough conversation, but eventually it morphs into something better - something more aligned.

If I hadn't had mold, I wouldn't have sold my clinic and dedicated myself to the online business that I have and love today. I wouldn't have experienced the splendor of Arizona.

I am now much less embarrassed about my illness and the messy parts of my life. I calmly teach people about toxic mold when they ask why I moved here.

Everyone has a messy life; lean into and grow into a better version of yourself. Create an even better reality in the upheaval. Choose what you want to leave in the past and what you want next. This book is meant to get you there.

PART I
DISCOVER

When you first suspect you have toxic mold, there is a discovery process.

It's not a joyous discovery like exploring a new beach while on vacation. It's more like being on a scary amusement park ride as you enter into a dark, ominous tunnel.

But it's important. In health and life you have to know what you're up against in order to create the best possible outcome.

In this section, my goal is to get you informed and ready for action.

The more information and support you have - from testing and learning to identifying your resources - the better you will feel about making big decisions. You'll be focused and clear, not guessing and second guessing.

I know this stage is intimidating.

These few chapters are the most technical in the whole book. Feel free to scan them if that's all you're up for right now! Your main goal is to extract what *you* want and need from this book.

1
WHAT IS TOXIC MOLD?

IN THIS CHAPTER

- What is toxic mold?
- What are mycotoxins?
- Where is toxic mold found?
- What leads to mold growth?
- Toxic mold in a historical context

INTRODUCTION

You may be wondering, why in the world does toxic mold exist at all?

But there are many historical examples of 'dangerous' things in nature that are designed to protect organisms: some frogs are poisonous, bulls have horns, and plants contain irritating sap. It is not known if the toxicity of toxic mold is to serve a purpose or is incidental, but it's sure potent.

Mold produces an array of toxics.

Not every species of the hundreds of identified molds are toxic to humans and other mammals, but some are. In minute doses, you may never notice them. Even in large doses, your health may not be obviously affected if you are healthy and eliminate mold toxins well.

Too much toxic mold that overloads your immune system and detoxification pathways can affect your health in a devastating way.

Learning is your first step to recovery. Learn at your own pace. If you feel overwhelmed or emotional, you can take a break. Congratulations on taking the first step.

WHAT IS TOXIC MOLD?

Mold is a type of fungi that produce multicellular strands called hyphae. There are over 100,000 species of mold. They need moisture to grow. They produce spores that spread through the air or are spread when you brush up against them.

You can see a mold colony, but mold spores are not visible to the naked eye. Spores can remain dormant without a moisture supply *for years*. Once moisture levels reach 70% (and sometimes less), mold can grow. Growth can continue at around 60% humidity. Temperatures for growth are approximately 40-100 degrees F.

Mold can grow with increased moisture, but mold spores can also spread when dryness increases, when the mold is stressed.

> "The period between 1960 and 1975 has been termed the mycotoxin gold rush because so many scientists joined the well-funded search for these toxigenic agents. Depending on the definition used, and recognizing that most fungal toxins occur in families of chemically related metabolites, some 300 to 400 compounds are now recognized as mycotoxins, of which approximately a dozen groups regularly receive attention as threats to human and animal health."
>
> — BENNETT JW, KLICH M. MYCOTOXINS. *CLIN MICROBIOL REV.* 2003;16(3):497-516. DOI:10.1128/CMR.16.3.497-516.2003

Not all mold is toxic; some are allergenic, some pathogenic, some non-toxic. There is an amusing category of mold called 'cosmetic mold' that is visible and unattractive but not toxic.

The toxins I describe below can cause serious health concerns, and are the focus of this book.

These are types of toxic mold:

- *Aspergillus*
- *Penicillium*
- *Fusarium*
- *Myrothecium*
- *Stachybotrys*
- *Bipolaris*
- *Gibberella*
- *Chaetomium*
- *Trichoderma*
- *Trichothecium*
- *Cephalosporium*

- *Verticimonosporium*
- *Monascus*
- *Petromyces*
- *Neopetromyces*
- *Rhizopus*
- *Mucor*
- *Streptomyces*

Stachybotrys is often referred to as 'black mold' and it also gets the reputation as the most dangerous of molds. While this could be true in a sense, *any* of the above molds can make you very sick. The most common molds I find on test results are aspergillus and penicillium.

THE ASPECTS OF MOLD THAT MAKE YOU SICK

Mycotoxins are the 'toxic' element of toxic mold that can be measured in consumer laboratory testing. These mycotoxins are secondary metabolites, i.e. by-products of the life cycle of mold. **However, they are not the only component of toxic mold that makes you sick.**

A water-damaged building, for instance, will produce a number of irritants to the human body that can collaborate in a dangerous synergy. This combines with man-made toxicants in the building, underlying health conditions and other factors affecting your health.

Please note that there are also other biotoxins, such as toxic algae, that cause the chronic inflammatory illness but this book will focus on toxic mold.

Some of the toxic components in a water-damaged building (WDB) include:

- Microbial volatile organic compounds (mVOCs)
- Beta-glucans
- Mycotoxins
- Cell fragments
- Mold Spores
- Hyphal fragments
- Bacteria
- Bacterial endotoxins
- Yeast

These are common mycotoxins produced by toxic mold:

- Aflatoxin M1, B1, G1
- Ochratoxin A
- Sterigmatocystin
- Zearalenone
- Roridin E
- Verrucarin A
- Enniatin B
- Fumonisins
- Chaetoglobosin A
- Citrinin
- Mycophenolic Acid
- Gliotoxin
- Patulin
- Nivalenol
- Dihydrocitrinone
- Satratoxin G
- T-2 toxin
- Diacetoxyscirpenol
- Satratoxin
- Isosatratoxin
- Trichothecenes

The total number of mycotoxins in existence may not be known. For example:

> *"(Trichothecenes) are a large group of mycotoxins that consist of more than 180 structurally related sesquiterpenoid mycotoxins."*
>
> — OMOTAYO OP, OMOTAYO AO, MWANZA M, BABALOLA OO. PREVALENCE OF MYCOTOXINS AND THEIR CONSEQUENCES ON HUMAN HEALTH. TOXICOL RES. 2019;35(1):1-7. DOI:10.5487/TR.2019.35.1.001

The Great Plains Laboratory tests for 11 mycotoxins that are emitted from 13 genera of mold. Vibrant Wellness lab tests for 31 mycotoxins from 7 mold genera (as far as I can tell).

To make matters more confusing, your home test results may not completely match your urine and blood test results.

In my opinion, the *types* of mold and mycotoxins are not as important as the extent of infiltration in the home and the severity of health symptoms.

TOXIC MOLD OVER TIME

Mold has been around about a hundred times longer than the earliest human life. Recently a mold fossil was found and dated at 635 million years old.

Our earliest ancestors appeared 5-7 million years ago, with humans 'like us' appearing only about 200,000 years ago and civilization as we know it only 6,000 years ago.

There are several references to mold, mildew, leprosy, fretting leprosy, and 'marks on the walls' in the Bible. Leprosy is caused by a bacterial infection called mycobacterium. There are even instructions on mold remediation, both for belongings and buildings, in the Bible.

This a verse from Leviticus 13: 47-52:

> *"As for any fabric that is spoiled with a defiling mold—any woolen or linen clothing, any woven or knitted material of linen or wool, any leather or anything made of leather— if the affected area in the fabric, the leather, the woven or knitted material, or any leather article, is greenish or reddish, it is a defiling mold and must be shown to the priest.*
>
> *The priest is to examine the affected area and isolate the article for seven days. On the seventh day he is to examine it, and if the mold has spread in the fabric, the woven or knitted material, or the leather, whatever its use, it is a persistent defiling mold; the article is unclean. He must burn the fabric, the woven or knitted material of wool or linen, or any leather article that has been spoiled; because the defiling mold is persistent, the article must be burned."*
>
> — BIBLEGATEWAY.COM

There is a reference to poisoning by grains containing mycotoxic metabolites produced by certain fungi in 600 BC on Assyrian tablets.

In the 3rd century, St. Anthony, an Egyptian ascetic who practiced long-term fasting, helped two noblemen recover from ergotism (poisoning as a result of a rye grain fungal blight) and the Order of St. Anthony was founded in appreciation.

The Order of St. Anthony grew to the point of having 372 hospitals that specialized in treating ergotism. How interesting is this:

"The sufferers would receive ergot-free meals, wines containing vasodilating and analgesic herbs, and applications of Antonites-balsalm, which was the first transdermal therapeutic system (TTS) in medical history."

Wikipedia (details of all sources at toxicmoldguide.com)

It's now widely thought that the 'possessions' associated with the Salem witch trials in 1692 were actually ergot poisoning as well.

WHERE TOXIC MOLD IS FOUND

Your interaction with toxic mold usually involves:

- Buildings
- Vehicles
- Food supply
- The body

Since you spend the majority of time at home, your home is the most likely to make you sick due to repeated exposure. But schools, workplaces, churches and more can also be water-damaged and potentially moldy.

Vehicles can also become affected thanks to moisture and carrying moldy items.

Food is another source of toxic mold, and a whooping 25% of the global food supply is thought to be affected!

Lastly, your own body (it's a moist place) can become a colony for toxic mold. Although it's normal for you to have yeast and mold in and on your body - your 'mycobiome' - colonization of *toxic* mold within your body can delay your healing.

Mold can colonize in:

- Nose and sinuses
- Lungs
- Colon
- Skin
- Brain
- Sinus cavities
- Bone

Pathogenic mold, one classification of mold, is a type that can colonize and cause severe, acute illness. Some pathogenic molds are:

- *Blastomyces dermatitidis*
- *Histoplasma capsulatum*
- *Cryptococcus neoformans*
- *Aspergillus fumigatus*
- *Aspergillus flavus*
- *Coccidioides immitis*

WHAT ENCOURAGES MOLD GROWTH

Humidity

Mold thrives with moisture, and an environment with humidity above 50% is one risk factor for mold growth. Some parts of the world are naturally damp or rainy. Much of the world now suffers with air pollution as well, which can synergize with mold toxins in a negative way.

There are many reports of water-damaged buildings in England and New Zealand. There are tropical wet areas like the Amazon and the Southeast Asian islands that have constant high humidity.

Here in the US, the most humid or rainy states are:

- Florida
- Texas
- Louisiana
- Mississippi
- Washington
- North Carolina
- California
- Alaska
- Oregon
- Alabama
- Hawaii
- Tennessee

Not every part of the state may be highly humid. And states that didn't make this list can still have moldy buildings.

I now live in Arizona and I've had no problems with mold in two homes. However I have two clients in the state with moldy homes. I have also entered two buildings here in Phoenix with old, cinder block walls and I was immediately affected.

I toured an old home in Massachusetts that definitely had it. I've had clients in England, Chicago, Austin, and New York City.

> *"The severity of indoor dampness varies with the climate, but WHO estimates that in Australia, Europe, India, Japan, and North America, dampness is a problem in 10 to 50% of the buildings, and Sivasubramani et al. estimate that fungal growth is a problem in 15 to 40% of North American and Northern European homes."*
>
> — ANDERSEN B, FRISVAD JC, SØNDERGAARD I, RASMUSSEN IS, LARSEN LS. ASSOCIATIONS BETWEEN FUNGAL SPECIES AND WATER-DAMAGED BUILDING MATERIALS. *APPL ENVIRON MICROBIOL*. 2011;77(12):4180-4188. DOI:10.1128/AEM.02513-10

Water Damage to Buildings & Vehicles

Besides humidity, water penetrating building materials is an issue. The materials, combined with moisture, become a fertile ground for toxic mold. Some of the spores could *already* be in that material, even if dormant. Others could be airborne or in dust and then find a happy home in your moist drywall.

Plaster, wood, and concentrate have the highest propensity for mold growth according to a 2011 study. Drywall definitely has a bad reputation for mold, as it is widely used, porous, and contains wood fibers. It can be affected by high moisture levels alone, and by flooding of any type.

Different types of materials are prime to different types of mold:

- *Stachybotrys* spp. grows readily on gypsum
- *Chaetomium* spp., Mucor and Aspergillus grow on concrete well
- *Aureobasidium pullulans* (an allergenic mold) grows well on wood

Water damage to a building can occur in many ways:

- Hurricane
- Tornado
- Snowstorm
- Wind storm
- Object falls on house
- Appliance leaks (dishwasher, fridge, washing machine)
- Faucet leak
- Toilet leak
- Plumbing break
- Poor ventilation in bathroom or any room
- Gutters not draining correctly
- Water collecting in crawl space
- Foundation crack/leak
- Incorrect drainage
- Windows installed incorrectly
- Water heater leak
- Frozen pipes burst
- Construction errors
- Roof leak
- Sewer overflow

- Tub or shower overflow
- Mold growth in HVAC system
- Building built 'too tight'

It was easy to rattle off such a long list and I'm probably still missing some things! A building's potential to have water damage at some point in its lifespan is incredibly high. Improper repairs can leave mold behind.

Here are some statistics on water damage here in the US:

- 50% of buildings have some kind of dampness or mold
- 98% of basements will experience some type of water damage
- 75% of water heaters will fail before 12 years
- 8.7 years is the average age of a washing machine until hose failure occurs
- 30% of schools had a plumbing problem and 27% had a roofing issue
- 45% of a survey of 100 US government buildings had a current leak, and 85% had a past water damage

Not every water damage incident needs to end in chronic toxic mold. Any issues should be remedied within 24-48 hours, or at least have the wet material removed in this timeframe. If this window is missed, remediation needs to be more extensive. You'll learn more about this later, in Chapter 3.

An automobile can also be affected by mold from transporting wet or moldy things on a carpeted surface or leaving windows open in the rainstorm. Keep your RV or boat interior dry as well! These need to be winterized properly.

Some clients aren't sure when or how they got exposed to mold when they find a positive mycotoxin urine test. Often there is a suspicious bedroom from childhood or college when they think back.

Agriculture and food storage

Lastly, let's talk about the conditions that can leave food moldy. Mold can develop at many stages, from field to fridge.

Crops can become damp and grow mold:

- Before harvest, in the field
- Just after harvest, during early storage
- In transport
- At the grocery store
- In your cupboard
- In your fridge

Some foods are intentionally fermented, such as alcohol, cheese and kombucha.

You can also be exposed to mold from consuming an animal that consumed moldy feed. That means your meat and dairy products are at risk, especially if conventionally raised.

Mycotoxins are not destroyed by heat, so cooking doesn't solve the problem. I'll cover how to avoid mold in food later in this book.

SUMMARY

Now you know that toxic mold is a real thing, it's nothing new, and you are potentially exposed in many ways. A few takeaways:

- There are many types of mold, and a handful are dangerous to humans

- What makes the mold toxic are the chemical compounds it emits
- Mold can occur in water-damaged vehicles and buildings and in foods
- Humid, stagnant environments can encourage mold growth
- Chronic moisture + materials = trouble!

In the next chapter, you'll learn how to assess your own home and body for toxic mold.

2
HOW TO ASSESS YOUR HOME & BODY FOR TOXIC MOLD

IN THIS CHAPTER

- Symptoms of Toxic Mold
- Inspecting your home for mold
- Choices in home mold testing
- Body tests for mold
- Related tests to assess health
- Deciding what to test

As you read this chapter, you may feel you have about every symptom - and you might!

Know that having a lot of symptoms, or having a very debilitating symptom, isn't a death sentence. There are many, many beautiful stories of recovery. But none of them are instant success stories; it will take time to unwind the damage of toxic mold.

Having many symptoms in multiple categories is par for the course thanks to the pervasive, inflammatory nature of

mycotoxins. The good news is that you can come back to this chapter someday and see that you have less symptoms!

HOW TO ASSESS YOUR HOME & BODY

Testing is very important to determine the extent of toxic mold you may be dealing with, but I think it's best to first assess through a survey of your symptoms and your home. This builds your mold knowledge muscles and sets you up for a better long-term outcome.

Self-Assessment of Possible Toxic Mold Illness Symptoms

As you assess yourself for the following symptoms, remember that:

- Any symptom can have a cause other than, or in additional to, toxic mold
- You could have only *a few* symptoms, but the ones you have are debilitating
- You could have *many* symptoms, but this doesn't mean you won't recover

1. Fatigue
2. Brain fog
3. Twitching
4. Loss of motor function
5. Muscle wasting
6. Depression
7. Blood pressure issues
8. Anxiety
9. Irritability/rage
10. Suicidal ideation

11. Chemical sensitivity
12. Lost sense of taste or smell
13. Low sex drive
14. Irregular periods
15. Missed periods
16. Difficult menopause/hot flashes
17. Insomnia/Night terrors
18. Infertility
19. Weight gain
20. Irritable Bowel Syndrome (IBS)
21. Constipation
22. Poor appetite
23. Multiple food intolerances
24. Gastrointestinal infections
25. Weight loss
26. Asthma or shortness of breath
27. Nasal congestion
28. Post-nasal drip
29. Shortness of breath
30. Skin rashes
31. Acne
32. Puffy skin
33. Swollen or sore joints
34. Craving sweets, sugar or caffeine
35. Frequent urination
36. Urinary tract infections
37. Headaches
38. Frequent colds, flus or respiratory infections
39. Chronic sore throat
40. Chronic muscle pain
41. Attention Deficit Disorder
42. Eye irritation
43. Mental health disorders
44. Vertigo

45. Drugged or high feeling
46. Sneezing
47. Dissociation (feeling disconnected to your self/surroundings)
48. Metallic taste in mouth
49. Light sensitivity
50. Tearing and eye irritation

We've created an online mold quiz as well. You can access it at www.toxicmoldguide.com. This webpage also includes all sources, chapter by chapter. You can also scan this QR code to go there:

Assessing Your Diet

Do you frequently eat any of the following foods? Do any of them give you a negative reaction from the symptom list above?

1. Any grain: whole or in a product like bread or chips
2. Conventional/Grain-fed meat (not wild or pasture-raised)
3. Spices, especially red chili, black pepper, and dry ginger
4. Herbal supplements, especially milk thistle
5. Dairy products
6. Cocoa

7. Oat, soy or rice milk
8. Fruit juice and dried fruit
9. Alcohol
10. Coffee or tea
11. Lunchmeat or salami
12. Nuts
13. Popcorn
14. Leftovers
15. Dog food - applies to dogs only...hopefully

The above foods are not guaranteed to have toxic mold, but they are all susceptible to it. It depends on the quality and handling of the product, but there's also a bit of chance.

I was skeptical that mold in food could actually get you sick until I prepared to interview Dave Asprey in 2018. I realized that many of the foods I didn't tolerate well were, in fact, also the ones that contain mold. These foods are often high-histamine foods as well, which us moldy folks don't usually tolerate.

My major problem foods are definitely alcohol and dairy. Beyond that, chocolate, tea, coffee, popcorn, tortillas, tortilla chips and grape juice have bothered me.

I don't advocate for giving up every food on the list, but be cautious when you purchase and store these foods, and avoid those that give you a reaction. I'll discuss this further in Chapter 8.

Assessing Your Home

Next, assess your home or other building or vehicle where you suspect mold. If you don't suspect a current building, think about a past place you've lived.

I have heard of several college living arrangements that have known or suspected mold, for example. One client's dorm building was later condemned due to its mold toxicity! I've also had a client who lived on a boat that was moldy. And my own two cars both developed mold from transporting moldy items.

But some clues you could have toxic mold include:

1. Indoor humidity over 50% (can be tested by a store-bought moisture meter)
2. A sudden flood or burst pipe
3. A slow leak in the walls or floors
4. A musty smell
5. Visible mold along window sills, bathtubs, etc.
6. Moldy spots that keep returning
7. Stuffy air/poor air flow
8. Film on the underside of surfaces like chairs and tables
9. Standing water around home's exterior walls
10. Overstuffed closets
11. Known leaks in bathroom/kitchen
12. Gutters with incorrect drainage
13. Incorrect yard drainage
14. Damp crawl spaces/attics
15. Roof leaks
16. Window leaks
17. Natural disaster such as hurricane, tornado, snowstorm, wind storm
18. Object falls on house
19. Appliance leaks (dishwasher, fridge, washing machine)
20. Faucet leaks
21. Toilet leak
22. Plumbing break
23. Poor ventilation in bathroom or any room

24. Gutters not draining correctly
25. Crawl spaces
26. Foundation crack/leak
27. Incorrect drainage from gutters
28. Windows installed incorrectly
29. Water heater leak
30. Frozen pipes burst
31. Construction errors
32. Sewer overflow
33. Tub or shower overflow
34. Mold growth in HVAC system
35. Building built too airtight

According to a recent report from the Federal Facilities Council, a shocking 43% of buildings in the U.S. have current water damage, and 85% have past water damage.

Unfortunately, you cannot detect if mold is toxic by smell, sight or touch. You will need testing.

These are the options I would consider:

MOLD INSPECTOR

This is a good option if you own your home and live where a mold inspector is available. I find that many people are just running a home dust test without using an inspector. A good inspector is a very valuable resource!

A good inspector will look for sources of water damage. He may also test air samples and perhaps test via taping or drywall samples. He or she will give you a full report of findings.

But this person is NOT a medical expert! He or she cannot advise you on what to do next for your health.

I found several businesses in my area by Googling "mold inspector near me." I also found several organizations that certify mold inspectors. Some of the training looked pretty basic, and many did not have an online directory.

This organization, American Council for Accredited Certification, seems to require more experience and does offer a US wide directory (see resources).

The National Association of Mold Remediators and Inspectors (NAMRI) also looks reputable and has a US directory, and possibly contacts in Canada if you contact them. (see resources)

A few great companies I have worked with present in my Toxic Mold Masterclass. They are the Mold Pros, Yes We Inspect and All American Restoration. You can access this class series, and the resources, through the book's resource page, www.toxicmoldguide.com. The following QR code will get you there:

EMMA DUST TEST

We ran this mycotoxin dust test in our own home. This is the company I used: RealTime Lab. You could repeat this test after remediation if you want to inhabit your home again.

The EMMA uses a quantitative PCR (qPCR) procedure for the detection of ten known pathogenic fungal species in the dust specimens.

I have not found that this company presents a fully understandable lab report. But all the species they test for are dangerous, so any positive result is significant.

ERMI TEST

ERMI stands for Environmental Relative Moldiness Index and it is a *research tool* developed by the Environmental Protection Agency (EPA). If you visit the EPA's site, they unequivocally do not recommend the ERMI for home mold testing.

The ERMI reflects a patented method called mold specific quantitative PCR (MSQPCR). MSQPCR is a DNA-based method for quantifying molds.

> *"The 'application' of the MSQPCR technology has resulted in the development of the ERMI."*
>
> — HTTP://FLIAQ.COM/EPAERMI.HTML

It was released in 2000. It measures 26 molds associated with water damage and 10 common outdoor molds.

By 2006, the ERMI was being utilized commercially by mold inspectors. But the test was never developed for home health assessment, nor large building assessment, and requires a very specific way to collect samples.

An advantage of an ERMI mold test is that it scores the level of your mold versus the outdoor environment, which can help you decide what to do next. I had a client run one at home and one at work with Envirobiomics.

One thing I don't appreciate about the ERMI is that it measures molds that are not toxic. I believe the premise is that the load of overall mold can be taxing, but I think it makes it confusing and misleading when only a handful of the molds tested are toxic.

The ERMI can potentially be used as a tool for mold assessment, but know that it is an imperfect tool and I don't think it serves well as a stand-alone home assessment, nor a post-remediation assessment. It *may* be a good test to run if dealing with a legal case.

For our post-remediation assessment, we used our original mold inspector. We sold our home. If we were to have stayed, I would have also run a mycotoxin dust test, but we felt it too risky to even try to stay.

MOLD TEST PLATES

I once thought this way of testing was invalid, but I've since learned of a company, Immunolytics, that seems pretty reputable and helpful at getting you some answers at an affordable price point. Their test comes with a consultation on your results, which I like.

Advantages of mold plate testing are the low cost and the ability to run multiple tests. So you can test certain rooms, your car, your workplace - wherever you suspect. You can even stick a mold plate on your pet!

Testing Your Body for Mold

In many ways, the testing and remediation for toxic mold in your body is much more straightforward than home testing. There seems to be no one perfect home test and you'll likely need to utilize a combination.

Body testing for mold has come a long way. In the early days, there was no direct test for mycotoxicity in the body. Testing was done indirectly, mainly via blood lab markers for inflammation. Dr. Ritchie Shoemaker also developed a visual acuity test called Visual Contrast Sensitivity (VCS).

Now there are direct tests for mycotoxins in the body. While these tests are not perfect, they are a fantastic advancement in the field of mold.

The Centers for Disease Control does not recommend any biological testing for mold, stating:

"Mycotoxins are metabolites of some fungi that can cause illness in humans and animals, primarily after ingestion of contaminated foods. Low levels of mycotoxins are found in many foods; therefore, mycotoxins are found in the urine of healthy persons. Mycotoxin levels that predict disease have not been established. Urine mycotoxin tests are not approved by FDA for accuracy or for clinical use.

CDC does not recommend biologic testing of persons who work or live in water-damaged buildings nor routine environmental sampling for mold.

Persons using direct-to-consumer laboratory tests that have not been approved by FDA for diagnostic purposes and their health care providers need to understand that these tests might not be valid or clinically useful."

> — MELODY KAWAMOTO, MD, ELENA PAGE, MD.
> NOTES FROM THE FIELD: USE OF UNVALIDATED
> URINE MYCOTOXIN TESTS FOR THE CLINICAL
> DIAGNOSIS OF ILLNESS — UNITED STATES,
> 2014. *MORBIDITY AND MORTALITY WEEKLY
> REPORT*. 2015 / 64(06);157-158

I want to react to a few items above:

1. Great Plains Laboratory *has* accounted for mycotoxin found in an average diet and has set parameters accordingly
2. It's true that mycotoxin levels may be evolving, as this is all newer science
3. The FDA does not regulate *any* commercial lab test before use, so it's a moot point

There are definitely imperfections with these tests, but I still think they are very useful pieces of the whole picture.

Here's more information on how these tests work and current offerings available. **Please note that these are the current options at the time of writing, and offerings may change and grow over time.**

MycoTOX Profile by Great Plains Laboratory

This is the primary test I use in my practice, and the deciding factor for me was that it can be combined with other helpful tests; the Organic Acid test (OAT) and the GPL-TOX test for non-metal toxins.

I have interviewed the founder of this lab, Dr. William Shaw, who developed this technology from an interest in identifying possible causes of autism.

The MycoTOX Profile uses liquid chromatography mass spectrometry (LC-MS/MS) technology which is basically measuring a specific molecular weight of mycotoxins. Here's some information from the Great Plains Laboratory website:

"For many of our compounds we can detect amounts in the parts per trillion (ppt) which is about 100-fold better than any other test currently available.

We are currently measuring 11 different mycotoxins in our test from a wide variety of 13 mold types (genera) including Aspergillus, Penicillium, Fusarium, Myrothecium, Stachybotrys, Bipolaris, Gibberella, Chaetomium, Trichoderma, Trichothecium, Cephalosporium, Verticimonosporium, and Monascus. Since each of these genera contain multiple species, the MycoTOX Profile is likely to detect hundreds of mold species.

In addition, all the results from urine tests performed at The Great Plains Laboratory are corrected for differences in fluid intake using the technique called creatinine correction. Failure to use creatinine correction can lead to a thirty-fold variation in the concentration of the mycotoxins when there is variation in fluid intake."

— GREAT PLAINS LABORATORY WEBSITE

The mold testing I recommend is a challenged urine test.

"Challenged" means that you encourage detoxification in your body so that you potentially push more toxins out in your urine. This can be done with a sauna or intermittent fasting.

It's possible to get a false negative if your body is just so depleted and overwhelmed that it cannot mobilize toxins. But I have only seen this once.

One mistake I made was that I did not test for toxins in the early stages of my illness. This left me without a baseline to track my progress.

With the same sample, we can also measure:

- **Organic Acids Test (OAT)** uses the same urine sample to test for *Candida* overgrowth, *Clostridia* infection, glutathione deficiency, mitochondrial defect, and more. These markers could all be affected by toxic mold.
- **GPL-Tox** screen tests for many chemical toxins coming from gasoline additives, jet fuel, dry cleaning, plastics, pesticides and more. When your detox systems are overloaded from mold, your ability to clear these other toxins can be negatively affected.

Mycotoxin Urine Test by Real Time Labs

This is also an at-home urine test. It uses ELISA testing for antibodies to mycotoxins.

This test detects 16 different mycotoxins, including 9 macrocyclic trichothecenes. The mycotoxins tested are somewhat different from the Great Plains test, and they seem to specialize in trichothecene testing, and hold a patent for it.

One advantage of the Real Time test could be that they offer direct-to-consumer lab sales in 26 states. Great Plains MycoTOX must be ordered through a practitioner. Personally, I prefer a client ordering labs with an experienced practitioner so they can accurately assess the lab results and create a plan.

Mycotoxin Test by Vibrant Wellness

This test is also a urine test that can only be ordered through a licensed practitioner. It measures yet another set of mycotoxins, and appears to be the largest quantity of mycotoxins measured.

It does not appear to offer the creatinine correction that is performed by Great Plains. I have not ordered this test myself, but I've reviewed the report and it looks great. The company also offers a selection of other functional lab testing for Lyme disease, food sensitivities and more.

The following five mold tests I don't rely on much personally, but I wanted to share all the options I know:

Mycotoxin Testing My MycoLab

This test above, by My MycoLab, is a blood test that measures antibodies (immune respondents) to mycotoxins.

From their website:

> *"This blood serum test is the most precise and accurate test there is for the detection of the body's reaction to mycotoxins, both toxicologically and/or allergically. With the 24 results of this test*

panel, 12 IgG and 12 IgE mycotoxin antibodies, a healthcare professional can then take the next step and start treatment."

— MYMYCOLAB

Mold Allergy/Antibody Test

A mold *allergy* test measures antibodies to mold spores. Testing for mold spores can be useful to indicate current exposure to mold (IgG response), or allergic response to mold (IgE response). I don't usually see this test run in regards to mold illness. I believe it would be more common as part of an airborne allergy panel.

Mold allergies would be more like the typical sneezing and itchy eyes of allergies. It does not mean the mold is toxic. It is possible, however, to have concurrent mold allergies and toxic mold illness.

MARCoNS Nasal Swab Test

MARCoNS stands for Multiple Antibiotic Resistant Coagulase Negative Staphylococci and it's a chronic nasal infection that can result from immune weakness. The presence of this infection can decrease production of melatonin, an important antioxidant for sleep and immunity. It is a common condition in mold illness.

This test can not only detect a MARCoNS infection, but will culture and identify mold, yeast and bacterial infections in the nasal cavities. It also analyzes the severity of biofilm and how the client would respond to various antibiotics based on the organisms present.

The company we use for testing is called Microbiology Dx out of Massachusetts. Tests must be ordered through a licensed practitioner.

We have an informative interview about MARCoNS with Dr. Yoshi Rahm on our blog and it's linked at toxicmoldguide.com.

In the current trend of functional treatment of toxic mold illness, MARCoNS is often treated last or not at all. It can be very stubborn to remove, and it's usually not the 'biggest player' in your illness.

Blood Labs for Inflammation

As I mentioned earlier, before mycotoxin tests were developed, practitioners relied on blood lab markers, mainly inflammation markers. I do not run any of these labs, but I'll list them below for your familiarity:

TGF Beta-1 (Transforming Growth Factor beta 1): immune cytokine - related to asthma, Neurologic, autoimmune - may be elevated.

GGT (Gamma-Glutamyl Transpeptidase): liver enzyme - may be high in mold illness.
VEGF - Vascular endothelial growth factor - a polypeptide important for blood flow - may be low.

VIP - Vasoactive intestinal polypeptide (VIP) is a neuroregulatory hormone that may be lower and may cause shortness of breath.

C3a and C4a - Immune complements that are remanufactured rapidly, such that an initial rise of plasma levels is seen within 12 hours of exposure to biotoxins, and sustained elevation is seen until definitive therapy is initiated.

Matrix Metalloproteinase-9 (MMP9) - degrades extracellular matrix (ECM) proteins and activates cytokines and chemokines to regulate tissue remodeling.

Melanocyte-Stimulating Hormone (MSH) - anti-inflammatory and neurohormonal regulatory functions - may be low.

Antidiuretic Hormone (ADH) - hormone controls the amount of water your body removes - frequent urination, thirst, edema, may be low.

Osmolality - is a test that measures the concentration of all chemical particles found in the fluid part of the blood.- may be low.

HLA-DR, genes - The immune response genes are found on chromosome six. Patients could have two alleles, copies of genes (for each gene, one allele is inherited from a person's father, and the other is inherited from a person's mother), out of approximately 10 possible, as part of their genotype.

Visual Contrast Sensitivity

This is a test that measures the ability to see details at low contrast levels and is typically used as a nonspecific test of neurological functions. Many factors such as toxicity and infection can affect your ability to see contrast.

Images are presented that the viewer assesses, similar to your experience at an eye doctor. There are a couple of companies that offer the test online and some Shoemaker-trained practitioners may offer it in their clinic. It is affordable or free.

My ex-husband and I took the test and both of our results indicated that we had no issues, so I found the test to be inaccurate in our cases.

Other Helpful Lab Tests

There are other labs that can be helpful in your recovery from mold illness. I will cover these in in a later chapter, but I'll give a summary here:

Blood Tests:

- Full thyroid panel with antibodies
- White blood cell count (WBC) with differentials
- Vitamin D
- Ferritin
- HA1c
- Fasting glucose
- Testosterone, DHEA, estrogen, cortisol
- Epstein Barr viral panel
- Lyme-related infections

Urine Tests:

- Dried Urine Test for Comprehensive Hormones (DUTCH) - adrenal and sex hormones, melatonin
- Organic Acids Test - Cellular health, Candida, Clostridia, glutathione levels
- GPL-Tox - chemicals such as pesticides, gasoline additives
- 24-hour heavy metal test

Hair Test:

- Hair Tissue Mineral Analysis - mineral balance and heavy metals

Stool Test:

- GI Map or similar - measures for infections & intestinal integrity

Scans:

- SPECT (single photon emission computed tomography)- damage by toxins and other factors to the brain
- NeuroQuant MRI

WHAT TO TEST

Testing can get expensive. It adds up if you:

- Have lots of symptoms
- Have very serious symptoms
- Have inconclusive results on your home
- Need repeat testing of home or body
- Have multiple family members who are ill

- Are also spending money on home repairs, a new rental, new clothes, etc.

I know how real the stress is of all the money that's being spent. I know it's frustrating that it's mainly not covered by insurance, that it's not your fault, and that you're spending money on something that feels like your mortal enemy.

I have many clients who have done lots of testing and more with various functional providers or on their own. Unfortunately some people spend years, even decades, without knowing or acknowledging mold illness as a possibility. **Though expensive, these related tests reveal what you are dealing with for more accurate treatment.**

Two things to know:

1. Your health MATTERS
2. You don't have to spend on everything all at once

When you are:

- Beat down by your symptoms
- Tight on money
- Lacking an obvious support network
- In an otherwise 'great home' or neighborhood
- In a specific life situation, like a kid who's in high school (I've heard that one a lot)

It's easy to negotiate with yourself that you don't need to move out or spend money on mold recovery. I am very thankful that my ex-husband pushed our own situation forward, while I resisted change.

It takes bravery, humility, creativity and tons of self-worth to tackle toxic mold. Do it. I promise that you won't regret it.

Know that you don't have to do it all at once. There will likely be a *lot* to do. Don't procrastinate for the reasons I mentioned above, or any other reasons, but *do* move forward.

For example:

- Move into temporary housing and then figure out your next move
- Test your home now, and your body a bit later
- Test your sickest family member first
- Test your weakest body system now, and another system later
- Get rid of clothes, but not your computer just yet

I know I might get disagreement with the advice above, but I think it's practical because I know from personal experience how expensive it all is, even if you are a solidly middle class American. You usually have to negotiate on your spending priorities, but eventually you'll get through it all.

I often tell my clients, "If I had a magic wand I'd run these 4-5 tests, but these 1-2 tests are the most important for now, and it's your decision, based on what you feel is best."

The tests I determine as 'most important for now' depend on the case! Is home or body testing more important right now? (I usually recommend home first.) Are gut or hormones more important?

As far as what items bring into a new living situation, be sure to read the upcoming chapters before moving willy nilly to a new home!

SUMMARY

- Assessing your symptoms, space and diet is a free place to start!
- There are many great tests now available for mold
- What to test depends on your individual situation

In the next chapter I'll explain why toxic mold is so dangerous for your health.

It's easy to want to ignore the complex problem of toxic mold, but ignoring it can lead to really serious health effects, even for the heartiest of humans!

Client Story –

Matt moved into a basement apartment in graduate school. A competitive athlete and accomplished student, he considered himself immune to any questionable aspects of the space. In fact, it was a point of pride that he was saving money and thriving in any conditions…until he got sick.

He happened to be attending chiropractic school, so, while he didn't suspect mold, parasites and Lyme disease right away, he did eventually find these root causes.

It took time, but Matt fully recovered (he did, in fact have resilient health!), and went on to specialize in the functional treatment of these conditions.

3
HOW CAN TOXIC MOLD AFFECT YOUR HEALTH

IN THIS CHAPTER

- Mold Illness Terminology & Related Health Conditions
- How Your Health History & Genetics Play a Part
- How Toxic Mold Affects: Hormones, Immunity, Digestion, Brain Health, Cellular Energy
- How Toxic Mold Can Lead to Chronic Diseases

INTRODUCTION

THE IMMUNE SYSTEM is designed to respond to threats through a host of agents that can identify, engulf and destroy attackers. Inflammatory agents are one of these weapons.

While you might think of inflammation as inherently 'bad,' a certain amount of inflammation is normal as you go through life's insults: stubbing your toe, staying up too late, eating bad sushi, or catching a cold.

When inflammation becomes chronic, whether through chronic mental/emotional stress, poor diet, lack of movement or persistent toxins, this is when things go haywire.

We'll cover recovery protocols later in this book, but for now learn some of the powerful mechanisms of disarray caused by toxic mold to your body systems.

MOLD TERMINOLOGY

Dr. Ritchie Shoemaker is an important trailblazer in the field of modern biotoxin illness. Beginning his career in 1980 as a primary care physician in rural Maryland, he became intrigued by a local aquatic biotoxin making people sick. In 2002, he began a biotoxin illness clinic.

He has published 11 books, treated over 10,000 patients and trained practitioners in his techniques. He coined the term Chronic Inflammatory Response Syndrome (CIRS) to describe the systemic immune-modulated response to mycotoxins that gets stuck 'on' in the body. If CIRS is due to a water-damaged building, it may be called CIRS-WDB.

There are other terms and cousins related to CIRS. These include:

- Chronic Fatigue Syndrome (CFS)
- Environmentally Acquired Illness (EAI)
- Gulf War Syndrome
- Sick Building Syndrome
- Chronic Biotoxin Associated Illness
- Dampness and Mold Hypersensitivity Syndrome (DMHS)
- Toxic Mold Illness (my preferred term)

Mold illness has been associated with:

- MARCoNS (a chronic nasal infection)
- Lyme disease
- MS (multiple sclerosis)
- Diabetes
- Heart disease
- EBV (Epstein Barr virus)
- Hashimoto's thyroiditis
- Candidiasis
- Parasites
- IBS (irritable bowel syndrome)
- Mitochondrial disease
- Cell danger response (you'll learn more later)

MOLD & YOUR HEALTH HISTORY

Health history can be an under appreciated aspect of mold illness. For example, if you:

- Eat poorly
- Smoke
- Are constipated
- Have allergies
- Already had a major health stressor
- Are under emotional stress

…you will likely fare worse in a moldy environment. But the equation is not as simple as a list of good vs. bad behavior.

There is a concept in natural medicine called the Bucket Theory, which is the idea that we all have a threshold of toxicity and imbalance we can manage before becoming symptomatic.

Your bucket size may have to do with your age and genetics (see below), and will be affected by your gut health, your work stress, your home toxin levels, etc.

An important point to remember is that you're not sick with 'just mold.' You are sick with mold in concert with every other factor in your health.

The longer you have mold exposure, your body systems can deteriorate, infections can take hold, etc. - so now you have mold + your health history + new co-infections + other biotoxins from water-damaged-buildings + the physical and mental stress of chronic illness.

Within the same family and home, you'll see a mix of reactions to mold - from negligible to severe - because of the mix of factors discussed in this chapter.

MOLD & YOUR GENETICS

The following are a handful of examples of how your individual genetic variations could play a role in your response to toxic mold:

HLA-DR (Human Leukocyte Antigen – DR isotype)

There has been much focus on a certain gene that, if expressed, can hinder your ability to identify mycotoxins: the HLA-DR gene. This gene, part of the major histocompatibility complex (MHC), located on chromosome 6 p-arm 21.3, if missing or poorly functioning, is associated with increased mold sensitivity.

Human Leukocyte Antigen (HLA) is the protein the HLA-DR gene expresses and is found on most cells in your body which signal to your immune system which cells are problematic.

Without proper HLA production, mycotoxins can be stored in the body, and, being a lipophilic (fat-loving) compound, they have an affinity for the brain. The body can also begin to exhibit autoimmune behaviors with an HLA-DR issue.

I have not run this test on myself because:

- It's expensive
- I was clearly sick and knew I had mold in the home
- We had other types of mold testing we were investing in at the time

It's important to note that immunity itself is compromised by the presence of mycotoxins. Having a genetic issue will likely affect your overall response, but you can get quite sick without an HLA-DR genetic problem as well.

MTHFR (methylenetetrahydrofolate reductase) gene

Another genetic variant that can affect mold detox is the MTHFR gene. This gene converts folic acid to folate and assists in glutathione production. Glutathione is an important detox antioxidant for mold.

COMT (catechol-O-methyltransferase) gene

COMT is a gene that supports methylation, one of the processes in phase II liver detoxification that removes organic compounds called catechols. A slow-functioning COMT gene can also impair mold detox.

GCLC (Glutamate-cysteine ligase regulatory subunit) gene

GCLC is a gene that supports glutathione production and an appropriate response to inflammation. A single nucleotide polymorphism (SNP) on this gene could impair your detox ability.

Although it's interesting to learn about genes, they are not the only factors at play in your health. They may influence how sick you become and how well, or poorly, you respond to different treatments.

The combination of elements needed to repair the body will vary person to person, and I think it's more important to focus on your actual symptoms and responses to treatment. We'll cover that more in Part 2 of this book.

THE TROUBLE WITH MYCOTOXINS

Mycotoxins have a very low molecular weight and most are lipophilic - tending to combine with or dissolve in lipids or fats. This is a problem as all our cell membranes are fatty, and certain tissues, like the brain, contain more fat.

One mycotoxin type I discovered, fumonisins, is hydrophilic, meaning it dissolves in water. This is trouble too, as our bodies are mostly water.

Some mold toxins are ionophores, which means they have both hydrophilic and lipophilic properties, allowing them the ability to both cross a fatty cell membrane and dissolve into any watery solution.

All this is to say that mycotoxins get around. And if you lack the ability of your immune system to tag them for elimination, or if your body becomes overwhelmed by volume, their toxic nature can inflame and damage tissue.

MOLD & YOUR BODY SYSTEMS

A fascinating aspect of mold illness, for me, is learning exactly how mycotoxins affect different body systems. This also helped me be kinder to myself and more patient and proactive with my recovery.

Mold & Your Liver

Your liver needs to work well to detox mold. Unfortunately, mycotoxins overwhelm your liver and make that difficult. Here's how...

For starters, mycotoxins increase inflammatory cytokines in the body. This leads to chronic inflammation, which is associated with liver disorders, including fibrosis and necrosis. Research also suggests a link between mycotoxin exposure and elevated liver enzymes.

One huge way mycotoxins overwhelm your liver involves your genes. In a perfect world, your liver would filter mycotoxins, and they'd be escorted out in your urine or stool. However, If you're one of the unlucky 25% with the HLA-DR gene, then your body doesn't produce antibodies against mycotoxins.

Instead, for those that struggle with detox, mycotoxins go through something called 'enterohepatic recirculation.' That means that rather than being safely ushered out of the body, they keep recirculating, causing mayhem in the process.

What's most startling is that mycotoxins increase your risk of liver cancer. How? Well, believe it or not, some mycotoxins cause mutations in a tumor suppressor gene.

Combine that inability to snuff out tumors with chronic inflammation and elevated liver enzymes, and you've got yourself the perfect storm for liver cancer. Even low levels of mycotoxin exposure can increase your risk of liver cancer.

While these truths can be scary, don't worry. I'll be sharing plenty of natural ways to get your liver detoxing well - so you can get that mold outta ya!

TOXIC MOLD & YOUR HORMONES

Sex Hormones
One chronic symptom I dealt with for many years while undiagnosed with mold was breakthrough bleeding. This is when you have some menstrual bleeding when it's not time for your period yet, usually around day 15-18 of your cycle.

This condition is usually a result of low progesterone production. This can be due to poor egg quality due to age, stress, malnutrition, or, yes, toxic mold. Unfortunately I didn't learn this for a long, long time, so I hope you are learning it a lot sooner!

In 2016 I ran my first DUTCH hormone test that showed I had very low hormone production along with probable hypothyroidism. My hormone production was at grandma levels, but I was 42.

This is one sign of mold illness: low hormone production. You can also have high estrogen, but in my practice I more commonly see low hormone production. This can happen for men or women, and can result in:

- Low sex drive
- Weight gain
- Man boobs
- Erectile dysfunction
- Infertility
- Irregular periods
- Difficult or early menopause
- Fatigue
- Hair loss
- Sugar cravings
- Mood changes
- Brain fog

It wasn't until about 2019 when I read *Toxic* by Dr. Neil Nathan that a big lightbulb went off about how inflammatory cytokines, increased by mycotoxins, result in low hormone levels:

> "...perhaps the most central effects created by the dysregulated outpouring of cytokines are those on the hypothalamus. The hypothalamus is part of the brain that controls the release of most hormones; it regulates the pituitary gland, which is known as the 'master gland.' These hormonal imbalances are directly caused by the effect of toxins on the hypothalamus."

Here's an example of how just one mycotoxin, zearalenones (ZONs) - a metabolite of Fusarium genus - affects hormones, shared in a 2017 report in the journal *Toxins*:

> *"ZON acute toxicity is relatively low but it strongly interferes with estrogen receptors and, as a consequence, affects the reproductive tract. Moreover, ZON leads to decreased fertility, precocious puberty, changes in weight of the thyroid, adrenal, and pituitary glands; alteration of progesterone and estradiol levels in serum, fibrosis and hyperplasia in the uterus, breast cancer, endometrial carcinoma..."*

And here's an example of the damage of T-2 mycotoxin, produced by trichothecene mold:

> *"Finally, environmental levels of T-2 appear to interfere with LH transmembrane receptor expression in human cumulus granulosa cells, while also lowering FSH-stimulated progesterone production.*
>
> — LAUREN TESSIER, ND. *ENDOCRINE IMPACTS OF MYCOTOXINS*

There are additional reasons why your hormones may be off right now:

- Intestinal permeability AKA leaky gut (inflammation, liver burden, immune disruption)
- Dysregulated microbiome (poor detoxification of hormones, mold and chemicals)

- Toxic burden on liver inhibiting hormone detoxification
- Poor nutrition
- Normal aging
- Overweight (fat tissue producing estrogen)
- Constipation inhibiting detox
- Lymphatic stagnation/poor overall detoxification

I spent several years specializing in women's health and fertility. It's not an easy subject to teach as *so* many things influence hormonal health, and it's our human nature to want a quick fix.

Know that there's more to your hormones than stress, age, or 'God punishing you,' which is how many women feel in the throes of a particularly violent period or hot flash!

Metabolic Hormones

Mold illness impacts your hormones another way - by sabotaging your weight. As we've covered before, mycotoxins increase inflammatory cytokines in the body. This chronic inflammatory state promotes insulin resistance and induces leptin resistance.

Leptin is a hormone released from your fat cells and is crucial for fat burning. Known as the 'satiety hormone,' leptin is what tells your body you're full. However, mold illness can make leptin's signals go awry.

How? Well, if your body is constantly bombarded by mycotoxins, it activates your body's innate immune system. Eventually, this damages leptin receptors, causing a state of leptin resistance. What this means is no matter how much you eat, your body never feels satisfied. Leptin resistance also makes it more challenging for your body to burn fat.

The chronic inflammation that comes with mold illness also overloads the liver, increasing your risk of insulin resistance. Plus, when your liver is burdened with mycotoxins, this damages your mitochondria, causing negative effects on your appetite and energy production.

Thyroid Hormones

Hypothyroidism and/or Hashimoto's are common with mold illness. Here are a few reasons why:

- The liver, an important site of thyroid hormone conversion, is burdened by mycotoxins
- Poor gut health (see below) can contribute to hypothyroidism or autoimmunity
- Low iron, common due to mold illness, can contribute
- Low glutathione levels, common in mold illness, can contribute
- Direct destruction of thyroid by mycotoxins

Mold & Your Immune System

Some ways the mycotoxins affect immunity are:

- Increased susceptibility to infectious disease
- Reactivation of chronic infections
- Decreased vaccine efficacy reported in pigs
- Immunosuppression via depressed T or B cell activity
- Suppressed immunoglobulin and antibody production
- Reduced complement or interferon activity
- Impaired macrophage-effector cell function

- Damage to receptors on the surface of macrophages, neutrophils and lymphocytes
- Activate inflammasome-associated innate immunity reactions in macrophages
- Suppresses immunity leading to MARCoNS infection and melatonin underproduction

This study done on poultry even found the immunity of offspring to be affected:

> *"The findings of the present study indicated there were severe immunosuppressive effects in progeny chicks as a result of exposure of their parent hens to OTA and AFB(1) either alone or in combination."*
>
> — UL-HASSAN Z, KHAN MZ, KHAN A, JAVED I. IMMUNOLOGICAL STATUS OF THE PROGENY OF BREEDER HENS KEPT ON OCHRATOXIN A (OTA)- AND AFLATOXIN B(1) (AFB(1))-CONTAMINATED FEEDS. J IMMUNOTOXICOL. 2012

Toxic Mold & Your Digestive System

In theory, a healthy microbiome can prevent you from developing mold illness. Here's how: (see resources)

You are exposed to mold through the air you breathe, the food you eat and skin contact. All these areas of contact host a barrier to the outside world - your skin and its microbiome, your respiratory system (nose, mouth, lungs) and its microbiome and your gut and its microbiome. Even your vagina has a microbiome.

Your microbiome, in partnership with your immune system, can engulf or break down the foreign, harmful material that is mold spores, mycotoxins, bacteria and cell fragments from food and water-damaged buildings that you learned about in Chapter 1.

You also learned in this chapter that sometimes genetics aren't on your side for this task, and your microbiome may not be either.

Despite specializing in hormones and detox, we sell more gut supplements in our shop than anything else. Peoples' guts are suffering thanks to:

- The Standard American Diet (SAD), replete with additives, processed fats, corn syrup, and pesticides, is incredibly damaging to the microbiome
- Pollution in our air and water is also damaging
- Stress affects our microbiome, often measured by SIgA levels in the gut immune mucosa
- Radiofrequency electromagnetic frequency (EMF) affects the microbiome (cell phones, etc.)
- Toxic Mold

As I mentioned above, a healthy microbiome has the potential to disable mold and mycotoxins, and you may never even know you were exposed. That's pretty great!

But if your gut is not robustly healthy, and most peoples' are not, and you have prolonged mold exposure, the gut will likely be further harmed by your exposure to toxic mold.

A messed-up gut is nearly inevitable with mold illness. You may develop:

- Gastrointestinal inflammation
- Intestinal Permeability
- Dysbiosis
- Candida overgrowth
- Parasites or other infections
- Irritable Bowel Syndrome with constipation or diarrhea
- Food intolerances
- Poor appetite or picky eating
- Bloating/indigestion
- Liver inflammation

Mold & The Brain

A frightening aspect of mold illness is its effect on the brain. The brain, the control center of the whole body, whose cells cannot be reproduced once killed, deserves our utmost protection.

The brain is susceptible to development of inflammation, degeneration and blood-brain-barrier permeability, which can lead to more problems, all thanks to the presence of mycotoxins.

As I mentioned earlier, mycotoxins are very small, very good at passing through membranes, and are highly inflammatory and poisonous. This spells trouble for the advanced functioning that your brain performs.

Symptoms such as:

- Irritability
- Depression
- Anxiety
- Poor recall
- Muscle twitching

- Poor attention span
- Fatigue with mental work

All point to possible mold illness. In addition, about *every other symptom* of mold illness can be thanks to an inflamed brain, such as:

- Nausea
- Low appetite
- Indigestion
- Low libido

We offer some free guides on the brain and digestion at briddgitdanner.com if you'd like to learn more.

Mold & Cellular Energy

One of the most pervasive ways that mold affects the whole body is by hamstringing the mitochondria - the energy producers of every single cell.

How you *feel* with mold illness, that deep exhaustion, that all-around *something's-not-quite-right* feeling - I believe that's the mitochondrial impairment.

This mitochondrial impairment can leave you feeling incredibly scared, literally scared for your life. I encourage you to pay special attention to mitochondrial support in future chapters if you are in this category.

Mitochondria are cellular components called organelles. An organelle is a part of a cell with a specific function. A mitochondrion is a shapeshifter, from thread-like to spherical, and it has a double membrane barrier and a matrix that contains enzymes, ribosomes and mtDNA.

Your mitochondria have their *own* DNA, different from your DNA, that is *inside* your cells.

A major function of mitochondria that I want to focus on today is ATP 'energy' production.

ATP is stored energy that is produced from glucose, oxygen and other ingredients through a complex sequence of steps by your mitochondria. The mitochondrial respiratory chain, or electron transport chain, is this sequence of steps.

Despite being inside your cells and then inside a double membrane of their own, your mitochondria are sensitive to damage, and they create their own oxidative by-products as they produce energy, as you learned above.

"The complexity of mitochondrial structure and function facilitates its diverse roles but also enhances its vulnerability...Several lines of evidence suggest that environmental exposures cause substantial mitochondrial dysfunction."

— ZOLKIPLI-CUNNINGHAM Z, FALK MJ. CLINICAL EFFECTS OF CHEMICAL EXPOSURES ON MITOCHONDRIAL FUNCTION. *TOXICOLOGY.* 2017;391:90-99. DOI:10.1016/J.TOX.2017.07.009

Here are some examples of toxins that damage mitochondrial function or production:

- Shiga toxin from E. Coli
- Trichloroethylene, an industrial solvent
- Mercury in dental fillings, lightbulbs, fish, industry
- Excess iron

- Mold toxins such as aflatoxins, ochratoxin A and macrocyclic trichothecenes
- Smoking & pollution
- UV radiation

Toxic Mold & Chronic Diseases

Here are some of the chronic diseases linked with mold illness:

- **Cancer** - As we touched on in the liver section, there is a link between mycotoxins and liver cancer. Mycotoxins cause chronic inflammation which can elevate liver enzymes and eventually lead to liver disorders. Plus, some mycotoxins cause mutations in the tumor suppressor gene.
- **Mental health** - Studies have found that people living in moldy environments have a much greater risk of experiencing depression, anxiety, and sleep disorders. Even a recent Psychology Today article outlines mold toxicity as a common cause of psychiatric symptoms.
- **Neurodegenerative diseases** - Dr. Dale Bredesen, a renowned neurologist and neurodegenerative disease expert, cites mycotoxins as one of the primary causes of Alzheimer's disease. Mycotoxins cross the blood-brain barrier and impair neuronal plasticity. Their neurotoxic effects are also linked with Parkinson's disease and ALS.
- **Asthma** - People that live in damp spaces have more incidence of chronic respiratory symptoms. One study found that infants and young children exposed to mold had an increased risk of developing asthma by age seven.
- **Heart disease** - Mycotoxins increase oxidative stress,

which is linked with heart disease. Research suggests mycotoxins elevate blood pressure and alter your heart rate. Aflatoxins are particularly troublesome for your circulatory system and can cause heart hemorrhage.
- **Diabetes** - Mycotoxins may also increase your risk of diabetes. One animal study found ochratoxins decreased insulin levels and raised blood glucose.

SUMMARY

- Toxic mold affects many body systems, so many different symptoms are possible
- Low energy, foggy thinking and mood changes are common
- Different people may be affected in different ways due to age, genetics and health history
- Left unaddressed, toxic mold can lead to serious or fatal health conditions

If you have someone in your life who would love to better understand what you are going through with mold illness, you can have them read this chapter!

For me, understanding *how* mold created certain symptoms gave me some relief and hope. If you know your enemy, you can outsmart your enemy.

Next up we'll cover ways to find support before you get into action.

Client Story --

I have come across several teenagers who were exposed to mold thanks to less-than-ideal living situations while in college.

The most extreme story was of a young man I'll call Mark. His dormitory was later *condemned* due to the extent of mold damage!

But at the time his symptoms arose, Mark and his parents did not know why this promising young man was losing weight, and could only stay in a darkened room eating a couple of foods he could tolerate. He had to use coffee enemas to produce a bowel movement and had to wear headphones to block any noises.

Mark's mother feared for his life on many occasions. Luckily Mark had motivated parents who took him to enough progressive doctors until they got some diagnoses (you'll always have several once toxic mold has eroded body systems) and some helpful protocols.

Slowly, Mark has regained somewhat of a normal life. He has not yet returned to school and can't spend much time on a computer. But he eats well, spends time in nature and has started to have a social life again.

If Mark's parents had not been proactive, his extreme toxicity and malnourishment could have killed him.

Even if your symptoms aren't as extreme, know that toxic mold is eating away at you! Staying in a moldy environment and ignoring your health is very dangerous!

4
NEXT STEPS & FINDING SUPPORT

IN THIS CHAPTER

- What to prioritize
- Managing projects
- Finding grace in chaos
- Assessing your resources
- Asking for help
- A daily journal exercise to stay grounded

INTRODUCTION

LET me compare toxic mold to...childbirth.

When you are getting ready to have a baby in our modern culture, most expectant moms plan like it's the Olympics and they need to bring home the gold.

- What should I eat or not eat?
- What is safe to put in the nursery?
- What is safe to put on the baby's skin?

- *What's the best birthing class?*
- *Can I still do yoga?*
- *Who will host the baby shower?*
- *Who will bring meals the first week?*
- *Who's the best doula?*
- *Which is the best birthing center?*

I could go on and on, but you get the idea. Moms know it's a big deal, and that their baby is very important, and it becomes an almost obsessive need to 'get it right.' There are books about it, everyone's excited and giving you gifts...it's a community effort.

And then there's mold.

No one gets it. There are few manuals. It's often not covered by most insurance plans. You're sick and worried out of your mind. **And yet recovering from toxic mold is one of the most critical things you'll ever do.**

So if you are feeling isolated and beat down, it's completely understandable. This book, and especially this chapter, is for you. Realize that there is a lack of cultural awareness about toxic mold, but you will travel this path successfully. Awareness is growing and, I promise you, you have more resources than you realize.

NEXT STEPS

If you've completed some of the learning, testing and assessment in the first three chapters of this book, you may have identified toxic mold. You may still be investigating some questions, but you know you have an issue.

The good news is that you are starting to know one of your causes of chronic illness. This can help you decide the best next steps.

This chapter is about making your plan and shifting into healing action!

CHUNKING IT DOWN

What's the secret to tackling any big project? Chunking it down. Chunking it down means breaking a big thing down into smaller, more specific parts.

We do this all the time - while planning work retreats, weddings, etc.

But, when it comes to mold, you may feel paralyzed, without any instinct to chunk it down. This is probably due to:

1. A lack of information about the subject
2. A lack of sense of support
3. The fear and anxiety related to your current life situation
4. The physiological anxiety, brain fog and exhaustion of mold illness

Nevertheless, it's time to chunk it down, my friend. The first step, according to a blog I found by Tony Robbins, is *capturing*. This means brain dumping all the things you need to do into a list.

Give yourself some credit that you've already done some things! You are reading this book - maybe you've already done some testing and made some habit changes. Put those on the list and cross them off.

There may be some additional things to do based on what you've learned so far. And there likely is more learning to do before your list is complete...we are only on Chapter 4, after all!

Lastly, the list will change. You may think you found the perfect new rental, but it falls through. You may think that IV therapy will magically make all your symptoms disappear, but it doesn't. This is a work-in-progress.

Pause to capture your ideas so far, and then use the rest of this chapter to help sort out priorities and resources.

PRIORITIZING

The #1 thing to prioritize is your health.

That applies to you and your family members.

You will want to prioritize what is easier, what is cheaper, what is best for your kids' social life, what helps you keep your job, etc.

I often get the question, "Can I start treating my body if I'm still in the moldy house?" or, "What if I can't move - what can I do to stay in my (un-remediated) house?"

Please be very clear on this: you cannot stay in a moldy space and get well. Yes, there may have to be some compromises as you make the transition to a mold-free space, but please keep any transitional time in the home to a minimum.

Don't fall into the trap of, "I'll move when (insert some circumstance that is 3-5 years away)."

Yes, there are some things you can do to lessen the health effects in the meantime, as you make your plan to move and/or remediate. I'll cover those in Chapter 5.

But as you answer the questions of what to do about the items on your list, I want you to hear my high-pitched but dead-serious voice in your head: "The #1 thing to prioritize is your health."

The symptoms of toxic mold illness will only increase over time as you stay in a moldy space or neglect your self-care.

These symptoms can turn into serious mental health disorders for your kids, Alzheimer's for your mom, and heart disease for your spouse. Some of these conditions will be irreversible.

While I don't *like* to scare you, I do *want* to scare you a bit because the health repercussions are serious and if you bury your head in the sand now you may seriously regret it later.

No matter how much or little money you have in the bank, no one likes to spend money on mold. Whether you're in a small rented apartment or recently built your dream home (turned nightmare), the price tag may be different, but it will hurt either way.

Yes, some people may have more savings or a higher-paying job, but once you are sick with mold, all those things could disappear.

Depending on the source, anywhere from 50% to 78% of Americans are living paycheck to paycheck, with about a 10% increase since the COVID pandemic. Even amongst six-figure earners, 18% of them are living paycheck to paycheck.

The average American has $90,460 in debt and 56% of Americans have $5,000 or less in savings.

Most Americans are not in a great position to handle a large, unexpected expense. So please don't think, "If only I had more money like everyone else, I could pay for this mold problem."

Everyone is in the same boat, the boat just looks different depending on your situation.

One thing I often say to clients is, "You have to humble yourself." That means that even if you never thought you'd be sleeping on a friend's couch at 52 years old, you might be now.

Life throws curveballs, and you need to respond accordingly to protect your family's health. The solutions you find may be humbling, and you may have to get creative, but it's important to find them.

Let's say you go out and come home to find your house has burnt to the ground. You wouldn't try to live in the ashes. Mold is tricky because your house is still standing, but it's become a threat to you, especially if your mold levels or mold illness are severe. So hard decisions must be made.

I struggled when I started to write this chapter, because everyone's solutions will be different. Unfortunately I can't possibly think of all the options that are available. But I did come up with a list of resources to get you started, and I'll share more of my story below.

I have also listened to the stories of clients and community members. I've heard some rough things - like a house that was finally remediated, but burnt down in an electrical fire before she moved back into it. I'm not sure I've ever heard a 'happy' mold story. It will always involve loss. But I DO hear happy endings.

I recorded some client stories in our Toxic Mold Masterclass, linked at toxicmoldguide.com, and they were super inspiring!

DECIDING FACTORS

What you decide to do depends on many factors:

- How sick are you and your family?
- What did your test results and mold inspection reveal?
- Do you rent or own your home?
- Are there some big life changes you've already considered, like moving cross country?
- Can you work remotely?
- Do you have good employee support benefits or not at all?
- Do you have a strong local network?
- Do you have a better network in another city?

FINDING GRACE IN THE CHAOS

We just covered some rational things to do like planning and prioritizing. Yes, please use your brain and tap outside experts to solve problems. **But you also have a heart and a gut that have their own intelligence.**

When a project is big, unpredictable and emotional, you have to have flexibility, trust and patience. I mentioned earlier that I had a good deal of anxiety on my own toxic mold journey.

Anxiety is something I've worked hard to reframe in recent years and it's finally going really well. But I did have a certain amount of trust and patience to balance out the worry. I think some of this was because I was too tired to overreact. And another really important thing, that I'm just now realizing as I write this, was that I did not let mold become my sole focus.

I still walked my dog daily, took my son to the park, worked on my dream business, and even made travel plans. Honestly, I could have chilled out more!

I'm glad I didn't lose my ambition, because it's tied to what I really care about. I did not let mold define me, therefore I did not put all the time into studying mold or 'fixing mold' in my life. **I learned when I could, as it fit into my schedule, according to what need I was facing at the time.**

If I needed to learn about mycotoxins and my belongings, I did that. If I had a urinary infection, I addressed that. If I was extra tired, I rested. If I was anxious, I sat mindfully.

In other words, I followed the flow of the moment. It's kind of like having an infant; you can plan all you want but in the end you just need to respond to the baby's needs as they arise.

Care for yourself like your own newborn. Don't force and stress. Make *only* the decisions that need to be made *right now*. Your body is going through enough stress; don't add to it unnecessarily.

Yes, you will experience many hard things. Take them one at a time and allow life to present you with options; this WILL happen when you surrender and allow it!

Allow that you will take wrong turns too and no one is really to blame. Allow yourself to cry in bed when you feel particularly awful, and then dry your tears and know you will keep going and improving.

RESOURCE SURVEY

Beyond finances, you will need to pool other resources. You will need time, emotional support, expert opinions, and help with labor and tasks.

Take stock of the categories below. What resources do you have? What resources do you need to find?

Experts:

- Local mold inspector
- Optional online/distant home mold testing
- Mold remediator
- Homeowner's insurance
- Independent insurance adjuster
- Movers
- Cleaners
- Air duct cleaners
- Therapist
- Primary care physician
- Naturopath with mold specialty
- Functional MD or gynecologist
- Functional health coach
- Nutritionist
- Massage therapist
- Lymphatic massage therapist
- Local natural spas
- Health optimization centers (offering IV therapy, compression therapy, etc.)
- Suicide or depression hotlines
- Employee Assistance Programs (EAP)
- Nurse hotline (see back of your insurance card)
- Human Resources department/Paid Time Off

Community resources: (for food, shelter, labor, emotional or financial support)

- Church communities
- Babysitters

- Neighbors
- Friends
- Farmer's markets and Community Supported Agriculture (CSA)
- Sports clubs
- Family members
- Fundraisers
- Online crowdfunding
- Community shelters
- Garage sales
- Thrift stores
- Bureau of Land Management (BLM) land
- State and National Parks
- Airbnb
- Vacation Rental by Owner (VRBO)
- Offer Up
- Craig's List
- Realtor.com
- Upwork.com and other contractual job opportunities
- Changetheair.org - resources & mold advocacy

Education:

- Blogs - ours is BridgitDanner.com
- Podcasts - one is Mold Finders
- Books - I like *A Beginner's Guide to Mold Avoidance*
- Facebook groups - ours is Mold Recovery Group
- Instagram - mine is @bridgit.danner

What other resources do you already have? What more do you need that I did not mention? I have a directory of more specific resources at the back of this book.

SHARING & ASKING FOR HELP

I want to close this chapter by emphasizing that you do not feel ashamed that you are going through this.

Yes, some people may not believe, understand or respect the issue of toxic mold. I didn't experience that at all though; it's not a given!

Yet, even though I was a health practitioner, I felt embarrassed to have this 'weird' problem. It only seems weird because most people don't know about it. But that is changing.

Did you know breast cancer used to be a shameful thing? We can thank first lady Betty Ford for bringing it into the light with her 1974 diagnosis and full mastectomy that she shared publicly. Now we all wear pink ribbons and rally behind breast cancer awareness.

"In obituaries prior to the 1950s and 1960s, women who died from breast cancer were often listed as dying from 'a prolonged disease' or 'a woman's disease,' " says Tasha Dubriwny, an assistant professor of communication and women's and gender studies at Texas A&M University, in College Station. "Breast cancer wasn't even named as the onus."

Ford's candor brought breast cancer into the public sphere. After her diagnosis and treatment, the number of women getting breast exams increased dramatically, as did the number of women willing to talk about their own diagnoses. The silence around the disease had ended—thanks in large part to Ford."

— CORINNA WU. A LEADING LADY. *CANCER TODAY*. 2012

Confidently explain your story as needed, or skip it if you don't want to get into it that day or with that person. People can be a little resistant or confused by new things. This isn't a judgment on you. It's up to you to get your needs met in this world, and there *will* be people who support you. Find those people.

I am really thankful for my parents, who not only let us stay in their home but agreed to watch an hour-long lecture on toxic mold I had found. They were so sympathetic and so proud of us for all we did to get better.

The first step toward being treated well is to be kind to yourself. Set that bar of how you want to be treated by treating yourself that way first. Generally, people will match your vibration and, if they don't, just let them go.

When money is involved, people can get mean. This is why so many people struggle with their insurance, landlords and HOA. Again, don't take this as a personal attack. Ignorance paired with a fear of losing money is a dangerous combination.

Sometimes it's honestly not worth it to fight these battles. Your health is already suffering and you likely need to move. You need to think about the most important end goals and not get too caught up in 'righting wrongs.'

Try This Exercise

The following three questions can make your life a lot simpler. You may want to answer them in a journal as you start your day.

1 What is best for the health of me and my family?

2 What step do I need to take today?

3 How can I approach this step with ease and grace?

I recently heard a lecture by Doug Brackmann, co-author of *Driven: Understanding and Harnessing the Genetic Gifts Shared by Entrepreneurs, Navy SEALs, Pro Athletes, and Maybe You*. He said two things that really struck me:

1. You need to be able to hold yourself in the midst of your fears or you'll get sick.
2. You can see the external world as a nurturing, safe place.

I'm paraphrasing, but these statements were so profound for me.

It's your feminine nature that can *hold space* for your tender feelings. And you can look at the world as a world that *wants* to help you and lift you up. Guess what happens when you look at it that way? It happens!

Doug also said that this feminine bravery of being with our feelings is what *allows* us to get into aligned action.

SUMMARY

- Make a big project less stressful by chunking it down
- Always prioritize your health
- Accept blessings; go with the flow
- Don't be ashamed of what you're going through
- Identify resources and creative opportunities that exist
- Ask for help; you deserve a helping hand sometimes!

So now that you've embraced your feelings, identified your resources, and made some decisions about what's in your best interest, let's get into action in section two of this book!

Client Story –

Jeannie got hit hard with symptoms when moving back to the family farmhouse. She didn't know mold was involved for a year or two. A generous uncle took her into his home, where she was mostly bed-bound. She had to wear a mask when out due to extreme chemical sensitivities.

Jeannie found a handful of local helpful practitioners and got by the best she could, considering she couldn't work much. She looked what she could for free online, including resources she found when on my website - I focused on female hormones!

She relied on her faith and kept some creative projects going as her energy allowed. She tapped into the inner strength she has developed living as a modern woman of color.

As she's gotten stronger, she's been able to take on new work projects in the arts and can afford more testing and supplements. She's in a group hormone training program and becoming an expert!

She's still chemically sensitive and has had to move many times. But she has been so graceful and productive in this period of mold.

PART II
DO

Now that you've tested, assessed and learned, it's time to get into action. In the section, we'll discuss action to take regarding your home and action to assist your body in healing.

Action without intention is reckless. By now I hope you have:

- Gathered enough information to make good decisions about your home
- Identified local resources, from friends to professionals
- Prioritized what to do first

Inaction can *also* be reckless! By now I hope you have:

- Set dates on when certain things should be done
- Prioritized your health over convenience or pride
- Gotten support to move forward if you've too tired, tight on funds, etc.

Remember to hold space for your feelings, journal about what to do next, and take aligned action. Try the daily journal prompt from Chapter 4. You've got this!

5
WHAT TO DO ABOUT YOUR HOME & BELONGINGS

IN THIS CHAPTER

- Tips for when you're moving or remediating
- Investigating a current or potential home
- Managing humidity
- Sorting your stuff
- Legal issues in mold
- Scenarios for renters vs. owners
- How to choose a remediator
- Buying new stuff

INTRODUCTION

IN THE LAST CHAPTER, I gave you some practices and community resources that will serve you. In this chapter, we'll get into the nitty gritty of the decisions on 'stuff and places.'

First, a disclaimer:

I am not a building biologist, mold inspector or remediator.

I am a health practitioner who knows a little bit about mold remediation because I went through it, have talked to some clients about it, and have interviewed some great experts about it.

Because the *environment* is such a critical element of this *environmental* illness, this chapter is here to get you started.

I would recommend you consult various sources. This may be a mix of:

- Friends who've been through it
- Local inspectors
- Regional or nationwide remediators
- Online experts
- Books
- Blogs
- Chat groups
- Attorneys

You want to feel good about the decisions you make by being as informed as possible.

MOVING 101

I was surprised to find that more Americans own a home than rent, with about ⅔ of homes being owned. Younger people are more likely to rent, and children are more often living in rental homes. I was happy to read that there is a good racial mix among US homeowners, and that most renters report adequate conditions.

What to Do if You're Renting a Moldy Property

But, some renters did report heating issues, rodents, leaks and mold. Eight million renters reported some sort of leak in a 2019 American Housing Survey with 1.9 million reporting actual mold.

If you are a renter with a water damage problem that is chronic or was not addressed quickly, it's likely best to move. Some rental agreements now have you sign a mold clause that the owner is not responsible for mold and it's up to the renter to ventilate properly.

All of us should definitely run our bathroom fans, open windows and perhaps have a dehumidifier, but some problems are more structural and not the renter's fault (see legal section below).

Some owners may be very responsive to make the necessary repairs, and others not at all. Others will not remediate properly, such as just painting over a water damaged area with fungicide paint.

Even after remediation you may not feel well. **So it's better to move, and hopefully you can break your lease for medical reasons.**

If you move to another rental property, look through the building assessment questionnaire above, and ask questions about the property. You may be able to add a clause that you can move out if your health is affected.

What to Do if You Own a Moldy Home

If you own a home you will have to remediate for water damage. But you may not want to move back into it. For us, our mold was so widespread and we were so sick that we didn't feel confident. We would have been paranoid.

That being said, we did a great job in the end of restoring the whole house and cleaning it, and we felt ok in the house in the end. But we hadn't bought new appliances, and that may have been an issue, or some other unknown issue. We did run a repeat mold test with our first inspector and passed, and we documented this for the new owner.

Some people choose to purge, remediate, clean and move back in. Others perhaps only have a single-source repair problem that is not as severe. These situations are all but impossible for me to judge by phone with clients, so I weigh in based on what I'm hearing, but, as I said earlier, it's best to weigh all the factors and consult with various experts.

I did a small survey on my Mold Recovery Group on Facebook, and most people moved out of a moldy rental, some remediated successfully, some unsuccessfully, and some aren't sure if it was successful or not.

I would definitely move out while remediation is done at the minimum, and have it professionally cleaned (all surfaces with a non-toxic spray or fogger) before re-entry.

Moving to a new 'permanent' house directly after mold often seems to end in disaster.

That sounds very negative - but I have heard several horror stories! Your health is still sensitive, you probably have some PTSD, and you may not be thinking clearly. And if you *do* suspect mold after moving in, what do you do? I suppose you can sell and purge again, but it doesn't sound too fun.

I'm glad that we didn't buy right away, and that when we did, we bought a newer home in a dry state and felt very good about it.

My ex-husband recently bought an older home in Arizona and was worried about it. He ran a mold test during the inspection period but the results did not return in time and the sellers were in no mood to extend the timeline in a hot market. He got the house professionally cleaned and ran a fogger and now runs an air filter.

In a normal inspection, you can ask your inspector to look extra hard for any potential water damage. You could potentially supply them with a moisture meter for the walls and a humidity reader for the home. If it's *not* a hot market, you may be able to negotiate more time for the inspection period.

Choosing Remediators

After you have identified mold, you'll need to do what is commonly known as 'remediation,' i.e. remedying the water damage/mold issue.

In Chapter 3 we talked about mold inspection services, and I would really recommend this before deciding what to remediate. If you are going to make a lot of effort to remedy one area, doing all the right steps, but there is another unknown area of the house still with mold, you will regret it.

This is just one kind of error that can happen with remediation! Let's gather some others:

- Moving moldy things in your car
- Moving moldy things from one area of the house to another
- Improper containment during remediation
- Lackluster cleanup after remediation
- Staying in the house during remediation
- Doing the work yourself when you are sick or unqualified
- Remediating one area without remediating another area
- Letting water damage 'sit' for more than 48 hours
- Choosing a contractor inexperienced with mycotoxin containment

You may end up needing a few different contractors for your home, and some will need to be 'mold-qualified' and others don't have to be.

We got three quotes, which is always a good idea, for our first step of removal of water-damaged drywall and carpet in the basement. The guy we chose was the cheapest, but he was also experienced with mold and did the tenting, air scrubbing and HEPA vacuum.

But it was not actually 'enough' as he recommended we move all belongings upstairs, and the basement needed much more cleaning and restoration before it was safe for our health issues. **It's important to realize that contractors are not health experts, and they may not understand all the details.**

Other contractors we hired were for:

- Removal and replacement of damaged floorboards, beams and all siding
- Removal and replacement of all carpet
- Installation of new drywall
- Duct cleaning and fungicide application (this is important before moving back)
- Deck removal and replacement
- Whole house cleaning

None of these people were mold-certified. By the time we had screwed up on the first round, we had moved out and basically knew all our stuff was toxic to us so none of it could be saved anyway.

Moving Belongings

I strongly suggest you bring nothing from your old house, at least initially, and especially if you had widespread mold or health issues. You can 100% contaminate a new place as the mycotoxins start emitting from clothes and other items.

Remember the character Pigpen from the Peanuts? He had this cloud of dust and flies that hovered around him. That's your stuff and mycotoxins, but you can't see or smell them. But after a while, you get sicker from the exposure.

Transitioning Tips

You may need to be in your current house for *a little while* and you may need to sort your own moldy items. But if this makes you sicker, have another family member or friend do the sorting. Here are some tips that can ease or prevent exposure and symptoms:

1. Take items outside to sort them in fresh air.
2. Wear a full respirator mask with filters (preferred) or an N-95 mask and gloves.
3. Have a few 'mold outfits' that you put on to work and then remove before driving or re-entering a safe space.
4. Shower and use a nasal rinse after handling mold and then returning to your mold-free space.
5. Take a binder supplement if you are feeling mold-affected. More on these later.
6. Diffuse essential oils like cinnamon or tea tree while sorting through moldy items. A diffuser costs about $20.
7. Open windows and doors for fresh air.
8. Do not haul moldy items in your car! Rent a truck or see the following tip.
9. Get a dumpster delivered; this was a lifesaver for us and was also used for remediation trash.
10. After a remediation is complete, the whole house needs to be wiped down or fogged. We used spray bottles of ½ vinegar, ½ water and 20 drops of Thieves oil/On Guard

oil per 16 oz. bottle. Or purchase/rent specialty mold formulations and foggers.
11. After remediation, duct cleaning with a non-toxic fungicide is also recommended.
12. I would *not* invest in a $1,000 air purifier for your moldy house. It will not fully protect your health and the mycotoxins will embed in the plastics and machinery and ruin it. You can buy this type of thing for your new, clean space for maintenance.

You get much more exposure through breathing mycotoxins than touch. So protective clothing is good, but wearing a mask is more important. But you don't want moldy clothes entering a safe space.

Remove your mold outfits and leave on site. Change into new clothes before riding in a car. Shower when you get home, and do a nasal rinse.

Assessing a Potential New Home

This is a great starting point if you are looking for mold in a current home or a potential new home. Most of these suggestions are free.

Use your five senses:

- Do you smell mustiness anywhere?
- Does it feel humid or stuffy?
- Do you feel lightheaded, tachycardic (heart racing), drugged or angry in the space?
- Do you see any visible mold or water marks?

- Can you see or feel a film on the underside of furniture?
- Do you hear any dripping or toilet always running, etc.?
- If you touch these areas, are they wet?

Common problem areas:

- Ceilings and ceiling tiles
- Baseboards, especially at perimeters of building
- Under kitchen sinks
- Around bathtubs, showers, toilets and bathroom sinks
- Around washing machine and inside the rims (always leave door open when not using)
- Dishwasher
- Basements
- Attics
- Crawlspaces
- Closets
- Outer perimeter of house (standing water)
- Gutters (not draining away from home)
- Windows
- Under futons
- Rooves (look for signs of damage)
- HVAC ducts and air conditioners
- Electric toothbrushes and toothbrush cups
- Books, bookshelves, filing cabinets and filing boxes
- Storage bins and storage units
- Under and around refrigerators
- Floor mats, carpets and drapes
- Around water heaters
- Cars, boats, and RVs (always winterize properly and use desiccants)
- Houseplants (don't overwater!)
- Garages

If you are looking to rent or buy, ask about previous water damage and how it was corrected.

Bear in mind that *most* homes will have prior water damage; things happen! So if you see some water damage under a sink in an apartment, it's not necessarily a deal breaker. If that apartment is also in a basement and smells musty, then it's a no!

As I look back to my own home, we could have noticed the following, had we been looking:

- Musty smell in basement
- Gutters not draining correctly
- Slight mold on baseboards of basement
- Recent water seepage into basement

But most of our mold was not visible - it was in the walls as a result of poor drainage, improperly installed building additions and improperly installed windows. We had some water penetration in the attic too.

Except for a dampish basement, our house seemed fine. But we should have been running a dehumidifier in our basement the whole time, and we should have checked for correct drainage away from the house. The part about the windows and additions...we never would have known without a mold inspector or if we had bought our own moisture meter.

Managing Indoor Humidity

If you own a home or are in a long-term rental that you suspect is humid, buy a hygrometer. This is a fun new word to learn: it's a humidity reader for the air - like a thermometer, but reads the humidity in the room. They cost $5-$20.

You can also buy a moisture meter. These can detect moisture levels in walls and wood. They cost about $15-$40.

You want humidity ideally at 40% or less but at least 50% or less *in every room of the home*. If you are above that, you can run a dehumidifier.

A dehumidifier *does not* fix existing mold issues or structural issues, but it can effectively keep humidity at a level that does not encourage mold growth. This may be a good option for a stuffy apartment, a home's basement or in a humid climate.

Dehumidifiers cost about $50-$250 depending on their capacity. These can be purchased online or at local hardware stores, as can moisture meters. Like I said about air purifiers, do not move contaminated dehumidifiers to your new safe home.

Another option, in tropical climates, is keeping windows open and running fans. Some buildings are not built to be sealed up tightly, and it may make more sense to just keep a breeze going.

Any appliance in your home can harbor mycotoxins, and appliances that house water can grow mold! Maintain your appliances well, and **don't move a dehumidifier from a moldy home to a new home.** Mycotoxins get embedded in the plastic and machinery of appliances.

Sorting Your Stuff

What to do about clothes, furniture, books, toys, etc.? is a tough question. The accumulated financial and sentimental value is substantial.

In my case, we got rid of nearly everything. I kept about five items of clothing, four pairs of boots, one box of important paper and photos, one laptop and one phone. *That's it.*

At first we did not realize the health issue of belongings in a moldy house. We moved everything from a moldy basement up to the main floor, which was a big mistake. Then we moved a small amount of clothes, toys and toiletries to our temporary home; also a big mistake.

The first situation got me much sicker, and the second made a safe space not so safe anymore.

We did try washing clothes with special mold detergent, cleaning the house well with essential oils, and using 'mold candles.' The cleaning would help temporarily, but the clothes still made us feel worse.

The test: stick your face into the clothing item and breathe. Do you feel worse?

The paper in books is great food for mold, and I was devastated to give away my whole collection of health books, except for one notebook that I put in storage.

I had bought a $2,000 desktop computer just a few months before we found the mold, and it got completely ruined. I cleaned it and put compressed air into it several times to no avail. Powering it up made me feel sick.

Some furniture and other items we sold. I suppose this seems morally debatable, but, unless the buyer is super sensitive to mold, it will be fine. *You* react to your own moldy things, but not everyone will. We never got any follow-up complaints.

Some hardwood furniture, tools and other items we put in a storage container, hoping we could revisit them and use them again. As soon as we opened the storage locker, I experienced mold rage. I think my ex saved some power tools, but the rest we sold or gave away.

Mold rage is a sudden, irrational anger when exposed to mold. You may also feel other sudden symptoms like a drugged, disoriented feeling, a headache or a racing heartbeat.

I think this storage container technique is a decent idea if you have belongings you hate to part with. Clean them before they go in, and then see how you react to them in 3-12 months.

Mold can grow in storage units, so use one with humidity and temperature control and consider adding a desiccant device. This can also be a good option for storing sentimental items or important papers that you do want to keep, but not in your safe home.

Nowadays there are foggers, sprays and services companies that claim they can eliminate mycotoxins/mold danger completely. I do have concerns about whether these methods can fully eliminate toxins to a level that is just fine for your health, so please judge carefully according to your own situation.

Items that can be cleaned 'easily:'

- Metal mixing bowls and utensils
- Ceramic plates, bowls, cups

Items that are very difficult to clean:

- Computers, TVs
- Appliances like refrigerators, juicers, air purification units
- Books, photos, magazines, papers

Items with motors are near impossible to clean. They have cavities where mycotoxins can get in and you just can't get them out.

All paper items are really impossible to clean. You can scan important papers or keep them in a Rubbermaid to open only when really necessary.

Idea: You can buy a stand-alone scanner with a feeder and hire someone on Craig's List to input and label everything on your computer.

If you aren't used to hiring people you may feel this is unnecessary, 'weak' or that you can't trust a stranger. I challenge you to think outside your assumptions. As someone who has done a lot of hiring for a lot of various jobs, I know how helpful it is.

Items that 'maybe' could be cleaned:

- Clothes and shoes
- Linens
- Toys
- Furniture

This is my list of items that could potentially be cleaned with special mold laundry washes, non-toxic mold foggers with enzymes, or in a DIY 'mold bath' of vinegar, water and essential oils. I also see some people in chat groups using Borax.

As I said earlier, we didn't end up keeping any of this stuff, except for about ten items. Clothes harbor mycotoxins. I managed to rescue about 4 pants, 2 boots and have 1 notebook in a Tupperware box.

We put some solid wood furniture in storage to evaluate later. We got rid of all of it. We were clearly mold affected by our storage unit, and the furniture that once seemed 'valuable' now just seemed like random stuff that could be replaced. Putting it away for a little while made the decision easier.

Cleaning Mold - What are Your Options?

As I said, cleaning mold ain't easy. That's why we tossed almost everything. However, I totally get that there'll be certain belongings that are painful to let go. That's where the cleaning piece comes in.

- **Distilled white vinegar** - Vinegar is highly acidic, and studies have shown it kills 82% of mold species. It's most effective undiluted, except for fabric items. For moldy clothing, try soaking them in a 50/50 solution of white vinegar and water overnight. Then wash them regularly the following day.
- **Baking soda** - Sodium bicarbonate has a high pH, which inhibits the growth and survival of mold. It works great as a combo with vinegar. Try adding a ½ cup as a laundry booster.
- **Borax** - Like baking soda, Borax has a high pH that inhibits mold growth. After soaking your moldy clothing in vinegar overnight, you can use Borax as a laundry detergent for extra oomph.
- **Tea tree oil** - Has antimicrobial properties that can help remove mold. Try making your own DIY cleaning solution with 2 tsp of tea tree oil and 2 cups vinegar. You can also add a few drops of tea tree oil to the washing machine during the rinse cycle.

Trying a combo of the ingredients above will yield better results than just sticking to one.

I used a homemade spray with ½ vinegar, ½ water and 20 drops of On Guard essential oil blend in a 32 oz. spray bottle.

As far as clothing, if you want to go the easy route, there are some laundry additives specially designed for mold removal. Micro Balance's EC3 laundry additive is the one I'd recommend. It contains zero chemicals and is made with a mix of essential oils designed to rinse away mold spores.

What about dry-clean-only items? Some claim that the heat and solvents from dry cleaning vaporize mold spores. While I can't confirm this, I recommend finding a dry cleaner that specializes in mold treatment.

Tips Before You Clean:

- It's important to protect yourself when you're cleaning mold. That means wearing rubber gloves, a breathing mask, and even goggles. Safety first.
- Before cleaning any items, take them outside and brush the excess mold spores off to avoid further contamination.
- When washing moldy clothing, always use the hottest setting possible according to the care instructions.

Cleaning Mold No-no's:

- NEVER combine bleach with vinegar! Mixing these two creates a potentially lethal chlorine gas.
- Don't think you can clean *everything*. Be selective about what to salvage. Mold spores are incredibly difficult to remove, and you sure don't want to re-contaminate your newly clean space.

When to Hire a Professional:

If mold illness has left you spent and just the idea of cleaning your belongings is exhausting, do yourself a favor and hire some help.

Many of the very same professional mold remediation services will also clean household items as an add-on. The upside is that they'll keep the mold contained, and you won't risk additional exposure. The downside is they'll likely use chemicals.

To avoid this, you can also hire a professional cleaning service to clean your items and provide them with the natural products you'd like them to use.

SHOPPING

Replacing things is expensive, and this is also a process I'd suggest taking slowly.

You may want to start with temporary furnishings; this keeps you mobile and out of quick debt. Start with a card table, nice air mattress (let it off-gas outside for a while) and a few new outfits. Leave shoes outside the door. You could also consider buying an unfancy but comfortable mattress for now, and buy a nice organic mattress later.

I am a proponent of Goodwill and resale shops, but you do need to be careful. If you are *really* sensitive to dust and scents, it may not work. I replaced most of my wardrobe from donations from friends and resale shops. But more recently I tried on two things at Goodwill that gave me a headache.

Resale can be a good way to buy furniture too, ideally hardwood. If you buy a soft item, ask about smoking, fragrance and water damage beforehand.

I once bought a mattress for our guestroom off of Craig's List and we were running late. The guy's whole family was waiting in the car to go to church, so I hastily bought the mattress. It was so consumed by Febreze scent that I had to sell it.

I also bought a sectional sofa on Craig's List that ended up being scented, but luckily I was able to wash the covers and the smell settled down.

Asking friends for donations is a great idea, as many people are getting rid of things anyway and are happy to help. You can also utilize different 'free stuff' sites and Facebook groups.

You again may have to 'humble yourself' and not buy the couch of your dreams. Or maybe just have beach chairs in your house for a year!

Buying a new couch sent me into tears at a therapy session once. I was so afraid to buy something just to have it get moldy again and have to get rid of it. These are some of the emotional hurdles you will face in these trying times.

Another thing to consider with new purchases is chemical load. Synthetic carpet, pressboard furniture, shower curtains, new TVs and many other items will off-gas chemicals, sometimes years after the smell goes away. I will teach more about this in Part Three.

Beyond your mold sensitivity, you are likely chemically sensitive, so investigate the materials of everything you buy. Buy polyester shower curtains instead of vinyl, cotton rugs instead of synthetic, and air out any new items, including TVs, in the yard or garage for a few days at least.

INSURANCE

My general impression of insurance is that they will cover damage from a natural disaster or new accident, but not a slow leak, which they consider owner neglect.

Covered occurrences could include:

- Lightning strike
- Ice storm
- Burst pipe

You may not have a valid claim during:

- Preventable water leak
- High humidity
- Flooding while away on vacation
- Mold around a shower you never addressed

Check your homeowner's policy for coverage. **When buying a new home, look for caps on mold claims and the option to add insurance policy endorsement for mold coverage.**

If you have a sudden water damage issue, take pictures and act quickly to stop the flow of water, remove water and remove or dry water-soaked materials within 48 hours.

My in-laws got water damage from a heavy snowstorm and were diligent about filing their claim and getting their needs met. The insurance paid for temporary housing for two months and the repairs.

If your house is damaged by a storm, you may want to get an independent insurance adjuster. These adjusters fight for your rights as insurance companies generally want to pay as little as they can. It sounds like it can really benefit you in the end. See the online appendix for ideas.

LEGAL RIGHTS

I have not had the best attitude about legal battles as I've seen very sick clients who have, in my opinion, wasted limited energy on righting wrongs, and sometimes staying in a moldy home for years in the meantime.

But you do have rights, especially as a renter and an employee. You are entitled to safe living and working conditions.

I have one client who got a lawyer and is getting some compensation from her landlord for health and property expenses.

According to the legal website HG.org:

"If you are a tenant, and have discovered any mold in your rented premises, then it is the duty of the landlord to get the mold removed and pay for any such removal. Landlords, who fail to make their property free from mold contamination can be sued by their tenants.

Under the law, it is not the duty of the landlord to provide or pay for mold contamination testing. The burden of providing such proof lies with the tenant. But if there is, in fact, any mold contamination the landlord may have been neglecting his responsibilities and the tenant can recover any expenses relating to gathering of the proof, in addition to damages for any injuries the tenant may have suffered.

Mold has been linked to the following injuries and damages: medical expenses incurred on illnesses due to mold contamination; pain, anguish, and suffering; damages for lost wages; loss of

> earning capacity; and damages due to loss of companionship, comfort, and financial losses in case of death due to illness caused by mold contamination. Similarly, one may be able to recover damages for destruction of property due to mold contamination and, in extreme cases of neglect, even punitive damages."

While it may be best to consult an attorney, especially in an extreme case, also be aware of the energetic and financial expense of a lawsuit when making your decision. If you do intend to file a lawsuit, keep good documentation on costs and value of items, medical bills, etc.

As a home seller, you don't have to disclose resolved issues, only current mold or water issues.

SUMMARY

- Moving may be best, whether you rent or own
- Getting rid of items may be best
- If you own, you'll need to remediate or disclose issues
- Insurance usually covers sudden floods, not slow leaks
- As you sort through your items, practice caution

In the following chapters, I'll focus on some areas where I *am* an expert, and that's health.

Recovering from mold is not as simple as just getting it out of your home and body. Those things *are* important, but unfortunately it's not that simple.

You have a unique body burden and background, and the levers you need to pull to recover will be unique to you. You'll also likely have some mental health challenges, thanks both to toxicity and to the practical challenges of a mold invasion.

The finish line of the journey can feel elusive as well. It will take some knowledge and grace to accept that. Don't worry; I got you!

Client Story –

Paula was sick with a few severe symptoms for years before discovering mold. She had daily chronic pain, a burning sensation in her mouth and disembarkation syndrome- which is a kind of chronic dizziness.

She later discovered mold in her humidifier and behind bathroom walls thanks to a sloppy homebuilder.

Not feeling safe to stay in that home nor moving into another old home, she and her husband built a home in a new neighborhood.

The road to her lovely new home wasn't easy though- she lived in a temporary apartment during COVID which also had mold, apart from her husband who was fixing up the old home.

She's also still experiencing some symptoms, which may relate to brain degeneration found on her Neuroquant test. But she's feeling much better than she once did, and has a new home and healthy habits.

6
PREPARING FOR A SAFE & SMOOTH BODY DETOX

IN THIS CHAPTER

- Best order of detox
- How to open your detox pathways
- Pacing your detox
- Health conditions to consider
- Working with children
- Supplement safety & sanity
- Working with physicians and experts

INTRODUCTION

WHEN IT COMES to repairing the body from toxic mold, I find that people get overwhelmed with the volume of ideas, some with conflicting viewpoints and some very expensive.

A few traps people can fall into are:

1. Over-relying on supplements
2. Over-investing in one methodology or practitioner

3. Over-emphasizing the detox aspect
4. Detoxing too quickly
5. Expecting improvements too quickly

My aim in this chapter is to sort through all of these issues.

If you find yourself getting 'in the weeds,' you may want to revisit this chapter.

WHAT'S THE BEST ORDER OF DETOX?

I get this question a lot. While I think there is some merit to this question, I also don't think there is a simple, follow-the-dots detox plan.

Step 1: Masters the Foundations

I cover this in Chapter 7. As a reminder, have these things in place, or at least be working on all of them. Your body needs strength to detox, and the good foundations summarized below help ensure that detox happens gently and effectively.

The foundations are:

- Nature time
- Toxin avoidance
- Movement
- Quality relationships
- MATH diet
- Essential supplementation
- Rest and self-care
- Sleeping well
- Hydration
- Alignment to your values and goals

Mastering the foundations of good health provides these benefits:

- Providing essential nutrients to your cells
- Pumping your detox pathways
- Achieving the parasympathetic state of healing
- Lightening the toxic burden on your body

Step 2: Advanced Daily Detoxification

I am a big fan of daily detoxification. Besides eating well, enjoying life and getting exercise, we all need to give our bodies extra love to make up for the toxins we inevitably encounter as contemporary humans.

And, in the case of this book, you need that extra daily detox to support mold removal.

You have a lot of options in this category! That's a good thing. That means you can customize this step to your budget and your tolerance level.

I meet many clients who can't tolerate hardly any supplementation. And I have other clients who are quite strapped financially thanks to everything going on in their lives. That's ok. I find that everyone can find at least a few detox options that work for them.

Step 3: Targeted System Repair

The truth is that once you've been exposed to mold for a while, your body systems have taken a hit. I think the most surprising and disappointing part of the mold recovery journey is how long this can take.

I used to think that if I just detoxed, my health would recover. I have the opposite opinion now!

It seems to be difficult for the body to find the momentum to reset after a long mold exposure.

You can be a great ally to your body by getting to know what it needs and giving it exactly that with testing and targeted supplementation. There could also be some other need-movers, like taking extended time off work in nature, that could help you.

OPEN YOUR DETOX PATHWAYS

Most practitioners will agree to 'open the detox pathways' before attempting a deeper detox. This means you are:

- Peeing
- Pooping (1-3 X day)
- Hydrating
- Sweating
- Breathing (beyond the basics)
- Sleeping deeply (when the brain detoxifies)

How to Poop

We release toxic metabolites through stool, sweat, urine and exhalations. Of all these, pooping is usually the biggest challenge for modern humans.

Many Americans are constipated, and constipation can potentially worsen with mold and/or other infections, an inflamed brain, dietary changes and supplement changes.

Ideally you want to poop 2-3 times a day while detoxing, which is even rarer. To help stimulate more frequent bowel movements you can:

- Drink at least half your body weight in ounces of filtered water away from meals
- Take magnesium citrate 300-400 mg at night
- Move more often, for example short walks after meals
- Eat more fiber: 8-10 servings of fruits and vegetables a day
- Eat healthy fats like avocado, fresh nuts, hemp seeds, butter, wild fish etc. (as tolerated)
- Uses prokinetic herbs like ginger and artichoke
- Use biliary herbs such as dandelion and gentian
- Take a good broad-spectrum enzyme with meals
- Eat more slowly and chew your food well
- Investigate and address brain inflammation (see later chapters)
- Take probiotics, prebiotics or mucosal supplements
- Utilize castor oils packs paired with essential oils like peppermint

I have been taking a prebiotic, MegaPre, with my probiotic, Megasporebiotic, lately and it's really bulking my stools and I'm having 2-3 bowel movements per day. I also get more frequent bowel movements when I remember to use digestive enzymes at big meals. I use Digest Gold by Enzymedica.

I've also had improvements with prokinetic herbs like Mega-Guard and mucosal support such as MegaMucosa. I am generally not constipated though, except when I had a concussion in

2020. Your brain controls the vagal nerve activity that stimulates digestion. I was also nauseous daily.

After a concussion, I had to take a multi-faceted approach. You may need to as well. Constipation, which is a bowel movement coming beyond every 24 hours, is a problem that needs your attention.

My clients generally come to me already quite knowledgeable about health and experienced in trying many protocols, so my approach is more to meet them where they are at. If there is an issue with any of the detox functions above, we will address it.

Some practitioners have an order they follow regarding the removal of heavy metals, parasites, etc. Again, while these *can* be useful, I don't think they are exactly necessary for every case.

Most clients can't test for everything at once. So we are addressing what we *do* know via test results, and what we know from their signs and symptoms.

I was an acupuncturist for many years before studying functional medicine. I do love testing, especially in these complex cases, but there is still much to be said for an old-fashioned assessment.

How to Sleep

For example, if a client isn't sleeping well, we know they aren't sleeping well because...it's happening. There are lots of possible reasons, but they can overlap, and some of the protocols overlap too.

Testing may reveal:

- Toxic mold (urine test)
- High nighttime cortisol (urine test)
- Low melatonin (urine test)
- High inflammation (blood test)
- Brain area damage (scan)
- Parasites (stool test)
- Blood sugar issues (blood test)

But in the absence of all these test results, I can have the client practice management and sleep hygiene. I can provide some calming herbs like ashwagandha or supplemental melatonin.

A chronically ill person may have several factors affecting sleep. These will not all be fixed overnight. So addressing sleep directly is not *ignoring* root causes, it's addressing a vital part of detoxification and healing each night.

Which I hope is illustrating my point. The plan needs to fit the client:

- What are her worst symptoms right now?
- How well does he tolerate supplements?
- Is she in a mold-free space yet?

See Chapter 10 for sleep tips.

Pace of Detox

About 5 months after finding mold I interviewed a mold-literate MD on my podcast. The question I asked her, on the edge of my seat, was, "How long does it take to get better?"

I think she said 3-6 months, I can't recall, but I know it was way less time than it actually took me to recover. So I tend to tell people, "It's going to take a long time."

I'm not trying to be a downer, but rather a realist. If someone told you marathons were easy, so you signed up and never trained, you'd be enthusiastic at first, but after a few miles you'd be pretty discouraged.

I have yet to meet the easy, uncomplicated mold client. They are in this mess because of an array of factors. Maybe one could say that if you've been sicker longer, or extremely sick, it will take longer. That's about the only generalization I can make.

One thing I feel strongly about is: don't detox faster than your body can handle. That means if you are getting *any* side effects, you need to pull back.

Some side effects I experienced were:

- Multi-day headaches
- Nausea
- Irritability

Side effects generally happen when you stir the toxic soup inside of you with a new supplement or technique, and you feel worse. While this isn't the end of the world or a sign that you should never do it again, you should cut back or address it in some other way.

Examples:

- If 1 capsule of probiotic gives you loose stool, cut back to a ½ capsule every other day

- If 2 capsules of a binder at night gives you a headache, try 1 or another binder
- If 20 minutes in the sauna made you feel awful, try 5 next time
- If you parasite herbs make you bloated, add activated charcoal 2 hours later
- Raw foods giving you insomnia? Re-introduce some cooked foods.

Side effects means that toxins are recirculating, or toxic by-products are being created, and your body is not expelling them efficiently. So you are essentially *toxifying* yourself to push through side effects.

The tricky part is that you don't know a therapy is 'too much' until it happens. So you will overdo and get a detox reaction sometimes. Just respond accordingly by lowering temporary inflammation with tools like:

- Sauna
- Binders
- Water
- Phosphatidylcholine (PC)
- Magnesium
- Fish oil
- Ibuprofen as needed

A detox reaction has another name: a Herxheimer or Jarisch–Herxheimer reaction. When you are in the throes of it, people call it 'herxing.'

Herxing is officially caused from an overload of toxic metabolites, as antimicrobial or antibiotic therapy causes massive bacterial death in treatment of things like Syphilis and Lyme disease and its co-infections. But people now seem to use the term for any side effect of detoxification.

When starting any new supplement or therapy, start at a low dose or lowered time span or frequency (for example, sauna and hyperbaric oxygen), *especially* **if you know you are sensitive.**

I am honestly terrible at following my own advice on this one! I get all excited about something new and forget entirely, taking a full dose. Luckily I am not super sensitive, but I have had a detox reaction from chelation therapy and hyperbaric oxygen. I also don't stomach antimicrobial and antiparasitic herbs too well, but that's about it.

In Neil Nathan's book, *Toxic: Heal Your Body from Mold Toxicity, Lyme Disease, Multiple Chemical Sensitivities, and Chronic Environmental Illness*, he says he treats many clients who can only tolerate minute doses of supplements. But in his experience, they don't get well *slower*, just with less supplements. So that's really good news.

There are SO many ways to heal and detoxify. When a new client tells me they can't tolerate anything, I have a list of ideas ready in my head immediately. There are *always* things you haven't tried. Some people heal by camping all summer. Some stay in a dark room and do coffee enemas. Most just piece it together, little by little.

Find your pace and path. If you can swallow a handful of pills, great. You are one of the lucky ones. If you need to be a hermit to restore your health, fine. Just don't push yourself beyond your *own* limits.

What you will likely find is that you slowly get better in peaks and valleys. You may feel a lot better at first in a new house, but then worse! This may not be the house, but that your body is now able to detoxify some stored mold now that it's not exposed to new mold. Gently support yourself.

You may get a new round of inflammation for what seems to be *no reason*. I had this and it was so frustrating. I found a little cocktail of supplements to help (see the anti-inflammation kit in my shop), and really watching my diet and sleep is key in these times.

You may have removed the mold, but you still have a chronic virus or amalgam fillings getting you down. You may have some body systems, like the digestive, endocrine (hormonal) or immune system, lingering with problems because they became so damaged.

This repair takes time. Remember your wins as you work through them. Are you:

- Able to work again?
- In a new house?
- Thinking better?
- Able to exercise again?
- Made plans with a friend?
- Cooked a great meal today?

Don't compare yourself to everybody! Trying to live up to an imaginary ideal just leaves you anxious or depressed. When you put attention on what is getting better, it grows. I'm not saying to blindly ignore what isn't going well, just count your blessings, feel your feelings, and chip away at better health from right where you are now.

My own recovery was up and down. A new house helped a lot, but a big move to the desert was initially disappointing. Fresh air and movement help me a lot, but winters are still a bit challenging for me.

SPECIAL CONDITIONS

I can't possibly think of all the health conditions out there, so it's important to review your own case with your care provider as you decide how to pursue your own recovery from toxic mold.

Do take your underlying conditions seriously, and *don't* start intense detoxification strategies without knowing what you are getting yourself into.

A few years back we heard from an elderly woman who tried a probiotic we recommended.

This woman felt that the introduction of the probiotic caused severe bowel problems that landed her as an inpatient in the hospital. The probiotics may have been a tipping point, but I'm sure there were existing bowel issues; dysbiosis (bacterial imbalance), her advanced age (over 80) and probably some other issues.

So, to my multi-symptom, supplement-sensitive people, please be very careful to add things slowly. You can't always judge it perfectly, but do your best and seek professional advice.

Here are some special conditions to consider:

- Autoimmunity
- Bowel disease
- Genetic disorders
- Mast cell activation syndrome/histamine intolerance
- Supplement sensitive
- Injuries and physical trauma
- Lack of mobility or flexibility
- Child or elderly

WORKING WITH CHILDREN

While I don't specialize in treating children, I love it. They are cuter and have more potential than us adults! I love to see kids and teens recover from food sensitivities, IBS and mold to return to vibrant lives.

Though I'm not a pediatrician, one thing I have heard many times is that kids aren't little adults.

They are:

- More chemically sensitive
- Likely won't take pills
- Can't be in a sauna as long
- May be pickier eaters
- Need to feel their autonomy
- Need to have fun
- Usually respond better and quicker to treatment
- Often require less medical intervention than adults
- Prone to certain neurological disorders
- Prone to certain digestive disorders
- Come into this world with more toxic burden than previous generations

I was shocked to find a 2019 study, published in the journal *Environmental Health Perspectives*, on the toxic mold metabolite zearalenone (ZEN) showing crossing the placental barrier, demonstrating the possible risk in pregnancy. It makes me glad to be writing this book!

There are *plenty* of options for kids. Examples:

- Epsom salt baths
- Smoothies

- Powdered supplements
- Castor oil packs
- Shorter sauna sessions
- Red light therapy
- Cooking with mom or dad

Note: I have seen more than one young adult live in moldy housing while in college. Could this be a factor for you or someone you love? Grade schools and high schools are also potential sources.

SUPPLEMENTS

We offer a service called Case Review, formerly called a supplement review. It's a really valuable service, because the average consumer has a hard time deciding what to take in the sea of options. I find clients taking 20 different supplements, and sometimes they don't even remember why they are taking something, even though they have taken it for years on end!

More is not always better - I think the body can get overwhelmed with too much 'supplement information.' You can also get nauseous! I generally like to supply foundational, nutritional needs, and then focus on specific, current needs. You don't need to treat everything at once.

Experienced practitioners have much more experience with the pros and cons of different brands and formulations. We have created and monitored many protocols in our career and have observed the outcomes. We love providing this high-touch service that removes a lot of stress and wasted spending.

We also offer lab testing and lab reviews (of tests you've already run) which gives us another opportunity to create supplement protocols. And we offer a lot of supplement reviews in our free eBooks and blogs to help consumers make decisions.

You can find them at:

> bridgitdanner.com/freebies
> and
> bridgitdanner.com/blog.

Supplements live in a grey area where they are mostly over-the-counter, so they *are* a consumer item. I love it when people take charge of their healthcare, but know that buying supplements, especially for advanced conditions like gut infections and mold toxicity, may pack an unexpected punch, or not hit the mark.

If you are ok with that, cool. If not, seek professional help. You can also download my Guide to Side Effects at bridgitdanner.com under the "freebies" tab.

HAVE A PHYSICIAN & WORK WITH EXPERTS

Work with carefully chosen practitioners, and have access to urgent care and primary care physicians.

Even if you like to 'go natural' in all things, there may be conditions you experience that require prescription medication. You may be severely immuno-compromised.

I shared that my big downturn started with strep throat. An untreated strep infection can lead to serious neurological or systemic infection. I was negative for strep on my first urgent care visit, but every natural remedy failed. I'm glad I returned a few days later, to find out I had a raging strep infection.

Months later, I got the first urinary tract infection of my life. Again I tried everything, but I was in awful pain. The first antibiotic we tried was 'gentler,' and didn't work. I had to find an urgent care clinic while on a road trip to get a stronger prescription.

I once read a quote on Instagram that said, 'we heal with others,' or something like that! We can't really survive or thrive alone. We need farmers, construction workers, electricians, childcare providers, teachers, etc.

The same goes for healthcare: don't try to go it alone. Build a little team around you - we all need people!

SUMMARY

As you move into action in Part 2 of this book, remember to:

- Start new therapies at a lower dose, time or frequency
- Start one new thing at a time! (This helps to know what's causing what)
- Make sure your detox pathways are working before deeper detoxification
- Layer therapies and build them into your lifestyle as tolerated
- Remember that the most expensive therapy isn't necessarily the most effective
- Remember that relaxation helps you heal; prioritize it!
- Moderate your expectations on any new thing
- Have curiosity and play around trying new things
- Use your inner compass to make decisions
- Lower inflammation if you are Herzing
- Have grace that not everything will be the magic bullet
- Realize that nothing is the magic bullet!

Client Story –

My client Max got sicker and sicker, eventually leaving his job and relying on his family for support. Max grew *very* sensitive- to foods, dust, computer screens and driving.

Conventional physicians suspected he was paranoid. Alternative practitioners gave him supplements he couldn't tolerate. Max has to baby step his protocol like crazy. He will take a pinch of a supplement rather than a whole capsule. Any misstep could mean a 3-day setback.

Luckily Max knows his body, having gone through this for a while. A win to him is taking a supplement, however small the dose, without a massively poor reaction.

But meanwhile Max is having the mold in his garage treated and avoiding that space and its belongings. And he has been able to work again from home, though at a slower pace. He communicates about his limitations with his supervisors as needed.

My favorite part of Max's story is that he volunteered as a crisis line operator when he was bedridden. Having been through so much, he had a lot of compassion for others, and people would call and ask for him! It's such a great example of turning a mess into a blessing.

7
STEP 1: MASTER THE FOUNDATIONS OF GOOD HEALTH

IN THIS CHAPTER

- My top ten foundations of good health
- How to stay aligned to your values and goals during this trying time
- The foundations of a good diet
- How to eat food
- Essential supplements to ensure cellular nutrition

INTRODUCTION

IN CHAPTER 4 you read an overview of my approach to detoxification and healing. In this chapter, we'll cover all aspects of step one, mastering the foundations of good health.

The foundations are:

- Nature time
- Toxin avoidance
- Movement

- Rest and self-care
- Sleeping well
- Hydration
- Alignment to your values and mission
- Quality relationships
- MATH diet
- Essential supplementation

Although it's tempting to skip ahead to detox techniques, these ten items, dialed in on a daily basis, provide *essential* support as you heal.

Mastering the foundations of good health provides these benefits:

1. Providing essential nutrients for cellular energy & organ function
2. Stimulating your detox pathways
3. Shifting into parasympathetic state (needed for healing)
4. Lightening the toxic burden on your body
5. Feeling motivated, supported and joyful every day

NATURE TIME

You may be surprised to find this one on the list, but it's so valuable on so many levels, and often ignored in modern culture.

Are you getting outside everyday? Even if it's cold, rainy, snowy or hot, you can dress for the weather and get out during milder times of the day.

Nature time comes in many forms:

- Surfing, swimming or walking on the beach
- Trimming and watering your houseplants
- Spending time with horses, dogs, and other pets
- Taking a walk in a forest
- Taking a walk around the neighborhood
- Backpacking overnight
- Long-term camping in the wilderness
- Gardening
- Playing team sports outside
- Biking
- Doing tai chi in the park

Time in nature provides these benefits:

1. Stimulates a parasympathetic healing state and a good mood
2. Reduces exposure to chemicals and EMF
3. Provides oxygen to cells
4. Provides negative ions, vitamin D and calming scents (in some cases)

Make a point of getting outside every day, whether it's sunbathing for 10 minutes, walking your dogs, or biking with your kids. You'll be rewarded with greater calm *and* energy.

Generally speaking, outdoor air quality is better than indoor air quality. But if you are sensitive to pollen, you may need to pick and choose when you go out, as well as work on your immunity.

Nowadays there are many severe fires in the summers as well. If the air quality is ever making you feel worse, stay inside and get some exercise indoors and maybe sit in a sunbeam!

TOXIN AVOIDANCE

Toxin avoidance is so important in this day and age, and especially important now that you've been exposed to mold. You'll need to avoid mold, dust, chemicals and possibly pollen.

I will cover it in more detail in Part 3 of this book as we explore avoiding future flare-ups and creating your best life.

Once you've been exposed to mold you may be chemically sensitive (reacting to things like artificial scents with headaches or a rapid pulse) and increasingly allergenic or asthmatic.

Everyone in modern society needs to reduce their toxic load and practice daily detox, but for you these practices may help you reduce chronic symptoms as well.

MOVEMENT

Movement is incredibly important as well, and may be neglected, just like time in nature. Many of us have desk jobs and lots of conveniences that make movement 'non-essential' in our lives. But it is essential for your health.

Exercise supports detoxification in several ways:

- Circulating blood and lymph
- Supporting mitochondrial function
- Increasing oxygen intake
- Improving mood
- Improving insulin response
- Boosting immunity

- Getting vitamin D (sometimes)
- Reducing chronic pain due to poor posture, etc. (pain stresses the body)

When I was at my sickest, I had little motivation or energy to exercise. I just walked my dog. But then I met a practitioner who encouraged me to exercise and talked about the benefits of exercise for my mitochondrial health.

Sometimes I would go to the gym and literally only use the sauna; I would decide I was too tired to exercise. But I slowly started to do some circuit weight training and Pilates. Low and behold, it did help. **Exercise uses energy but it also helps create more energy, as long as you don't overdo it.**

Types of Exercise

There are lots of ways to move the body, and everyone has a different movement Rx. **Most exercise experts promote a combination of strength training, cardiovascular training and stretching.**

Find the combination of activities you enjoy to include strength training, cardio, and stretching each week. Be honest with yourself about the types of exercise you avoid, and do those things! Maybe you need to hire a trainer to teach you how to lift weights. Maybe it's time to join a beginner's yoga class.

Challenge yourself a bit beyond your limits. Not way beyond your limits, but slowly challenge your body to do more and do new things. The same goes for your brain - it stays youthfully adaptable when you ask it to learn new skills and visit new places.

Ideas include:

- Yoga
- Stretching
- Pilates
- Walking
- Jogging
- Kayaking or paddle boarding
- Tai Qi
- Qi Gong
- Dancing
- Gardening
- Yardwork
- Weight lifting
- Calisthenics
- Playing with kids
- Golfing
- Tennis
- Pickleball
- Cycling
- Aerobics
- Softball
- Soccer
- House cleaning
- Rebounding (this is using a mini-trampoline)
- Stair climbing

Exercise is better done frequently than intensely in most cases. For example, don't just exercise on the weekends. Get in some walks, postural exercises, classes or soccer games during the week.

If you are quite out of shape, fatigued, or struggling with weight or balance, start where you can, and increase very slowly. You may be surprised how steadily your ability increases, and along with it your energy levels and optimism.

If you tend to get sore and fatigued from exercise, *do less*, and try taking antioxidants before your work-out. One option is H2 Elite by Quicksilver Scientific, a hydrogen tablet to add to water.

REST & SELF-CARE

Rest is an underappreciated thing these days. And sometimes we 'check out' in an unhealthy way and call it rest, like binge watching TV or drinking nightly wine.

Rest can be:

- Taking a nap
- Laying down to close your eyes for 10 minutes
- Taking a leisurely stroll for 10 minutes
- Meditating
- Yin yoga
- Legs up the wall pose
- Listening to music
- Reading
- Taking to a friend
- Listening to a podcast
- Taking a bath
- Doing a hobby
- Sunbathing

Rest is not just sleeping. Sleeping is super important, but it's its own thing. Be sure you are *resting* everyday. We are meant to sleep about 8 hours, be active about 8 hours, and rest about 8 hours. That's a lot of resting, and you need it!

Self-care can be resting, but it can also be more proactive. Maybe you need to find a therapist or book a vacation. Maybe you need to say no to joining that committee, or say yes because it fulfills you.

SLEEP WELL

Getting a good night's sleep can be achieved. It may take hormone balancing, nutrient addition, detoxification and more, and it may change with your menstrual cycle and other factors. But it's a worthy goal, always.

When you sleep you:

- Detoxify your brain
- Repair and eliminate damaged cells
- Produce growth hormone
- Produce the antioxidant melatonin
- Reduce chances of sugar cravings
- Restore energy for the next day

We all need a different amount of sleep in a slightly different window. But we all need it, just like kids do. You may need more as you are healing. You may need more just because it's how you are wired.

Don't stay up late reading, watching TV or on Facebook. Those things are ok, but get them done earlier! I shared some specific sleep tips in the previous chapter.

HYDRATION

You need at least 2 liters or 8 glasses of water a day, and maybe more depending on the weather, exercise and your size. Nowadays getting in 8 glasses of water seems to sound like some kind of radical health goal, but it's actually just *required*.

I think because we are more sedentary, eating more often, and consume all kinds of sweet drinks, modern humans are disconnected from our own thirst and need for water.

Aim for a minimum of 8 glasses of filtered water a day, or 64 ounces. Another rule of thumb is to take your body weight, divide it by 2, and that's how many ounces to drink per day. So if you weigh 150 pounds, that's 75 ounces of water.

I know water alone can feel a bit boring, but it's important. You can have other hydrating things, listed below, but also drink filtered water. Good times to drink are first thing in the morning and between meals. **Drink minimally or not at all at meal times as it dilutes your stomach acid.**

Other forms of hydration:

- Fruit
- Fresh vegetables
- Electrolyte drinks
- Soups
- Smoothies
- Berry-infused waters
- Herbal tea

One thing I notice while intermittent fasting is how much more water I crave. I drink a LOT of water and don't seem to pee more often. Again, I think eating often and drinking sweet things often throws our urge to drink water.

As you get healthier, you may be able to experiment with time-restricted eating and you'll notice this too.

Since fluid intake supports detoxification, it's especially important in mold recovery to hydrate. Other factors are sauna use (hopefully) and increased antidiuretic hormone, which leaves you peeing more often.

ALIGNMENT TO YOUR VALUES AND MISSION

Values

If you've ever had coaching, you may have completed a values exercise in which you identify a lot of things that are important to you, and then create a top ten, with #1 being the absolute most important to you.

This type of exercise is helpful, as sometimes the things we value in theory we are not valuing in practice. When you identify what you value, and you see you are not doing it, you can figure out why.

For example, if you value health and you want to eat well and exercise, but you keep getting take-out and skipping the gym, you can figure out why. Are you too tired after work to cook and work-out? Ok, can you set a crock pot in the morning, and work out at lunch time? There are always solutions.

Feelings

You can also work this exercise another way round by noticing when you feel frustrated or depressed. If every time you see a mess left in the kitchen by your spouse or kids you feel a wave of anger, that's a message! Maybe you value supporting others *and* being supported too.

Can you have a chat with them about how it makes you feel to see the mess and create a plan? Can you learn to walk by it sometimes? Can you set a timeline, like all messes need to be cleaned up before I cook dinner at 5 PM? Can you get a second dishwasher, or a housekeeper?

This mold recovery will be a challenging time, but this will especially be true if you aren't living aligned to your values.

I encourage you to journal on what's most important to you, and where you're feeling frustrated. When frustrated, feel the feelings, but then separate from them to see what exactly is out of alignment and identify possible solutions.

Mission

While in the midst of a move due to mold, your mission in life may be less grandiose and more nuts and bolts.

Know that even if you had to put aside other goals for now, your new, mold-related goals matter. Protecting and recovering your family's health comes ahead of everything. It's what enables those greater goals to be achieved.

You may want to set little 'missions' at every step of your journey. For example:

- To sort through the attic
- To find a new home
- To sell some furniture
- To buy and try some detox products
- To schedule a weekend at the beach

Turn your attention mindfully towards your mission. Put all your care into it and stay present. This attitude will be much more satisfying than rushing through it with annoyance. Every 'mission' you complete gets you closer to your new, mold-free life.

I did not drop everything for mold and you likely will not be able to either. I still had a young child and two businesses; one I was creating and one I was leaving.

Your mission can also include things like:

- Spending quality time with your kids
- Taking your dog to the park
- Doing your favorite hobby
- Doing your best at work
- Researching a new career or city

This is a time of growth. Intentionality will make it so much sweeter.

QUALITY RELATIONSHIPS

I am an introvert, but I'm also a people person. I need alone time, but I also need friendships, laughter and someone to solve problems with. The extra isolation of the COVID-19 pandemic really highlighted for me just how much 'people time' keeps my spirits high.

For your long-term health, and for your mold recovery, you will need good people around you. Some of these people will be the experts you choose to help you repair your house and heal your body. Others will be loyal family members and friends who help you with projects or listen to you.

On social media, there is an emphasis on cutting people out of your life who are 'toxic,' but there's more nuance to it than just that.

There may be some people in your life who are truly toxic and need to be cut out, such as abusers and drug addicts.

But there are others who are not the best fit for you, and the relationship needs less time together, or a new definition.

I went through a divorce last year, and this instigates all kinds of relationship restructuring. I definitely need to continue a relationship with my son's dad, but I keep it minimal and polite. Even though his family did nothing wrong to me, I don't interact with them much so I can have more space available for me to create a new life.

This ability to reframe relationships was one of the hardest but most valuable lessons of my adult life. When something hurts, we want to run away. **But if we give it space and remove the judgements, relationships can shift into the new dynamic that first the current situation.**

Throughout my divorce experience, I deepened relationships with old friends, tried new things and met new friends, and hired several professionals to support me and shift my perspective.

I literally had three divorce coaches, all different and all amazing. I also had a life/business coach, a couple of therapists, energy workers - I pretty much tried it all. I read books and took courses to help work through my fears and remake my life. It was all 100% worth it in how much positive transformation I experienced.

If you feel like you have too much heavy stuff to discuss with a friend or ask a family member, hire a professional. **If you're not** used to spending money on yourself for services, step out of your comfort zone and try it.

As adults, we have fewer opportunities to make new friends, or so it seems. But you can join MeetUp groups (it's a free app), take classes, organize block parties, or join a prayer group - whatever interests you. You will meet like-minded people and new friendships will naturally emerge.

Adding new, positive people into your life is just as important as decreasing time spent with people who are no longer a fit.

When you are going through a crisis, you may feel guilt about being needy or being a 'taker.' Life has give and take. You love to help your loved ones when they are in need; don't feel guilty about accepting help now. Someday you can return the favor. For now, say thank you, give hugs, and express your gratitude in meditation and journaling.

EAT A MATH DIET

After getting lots of questions from my community about what's best to eat, I came up with my own diet, called the MATH diet.

My basic dietary principles are as follows, and then I'll get into more specifics for mold and food quality later in this book.

Microbiome-Friendly

Unfortunately, our modern culture is eating fewer and fewer foods. We are getting lots of calories, but they are mainly from pizza, chicken, dessert items, pasta, rice, alcohol, sports drinks, and soda.

Even if you try to eat healthfully, you may be in a rut because of habit or food sensitivity issues (see below). Or you may live in a place with poor access to healthy, fresh food.

Our ancestors, who foraged and hunted, got a wide variety of seasonal foods. They also didn't use hand sanitizer or take antibiotics! They may not have lived as long, but they had better microbiomes.

Our standard westernized lifestyle has been associated with worse microbiomes and many accompanying issues, including obesity and other diseases.

Get a wide variety of fibers. Buy vegetables you don't usually buy or don't know how to cook. Go to the farmer's market. Join a Community Supported Agriculture program. Eat some beans or lentils if tolerated. Eat fermented foods like kimchi or sauerkraut (you just need a bit).

I loved Dr. Datis Kharazzian's idea for a high fiber shake: go buy a bunch of different vegetables, like 12 or 15, preferably organic. Clean and chop into chunks. Mix together and freeze. Pour some into a Vitamix or similar blender with water and anything you like, including canned coconut milk, almond milk, raw seeds or collagen powder.

If you are not used to eating a variety of fibers, you may need to move slowly with the food portion of this advice, as your body may not yet have the right bacterial population to match those varieties of fibers. Proceed, but slowly!

Anti-Inflammatory

Foods *to avoid* that cause inflammation include:

- Dairy (all mammal dairy)
- Sugar
- Wheat
- Alcohol
- Factory-farmed meats
- Processed fats like canola oil or margarine
- Non-organic cereals and produce
- Processed foods like muffins, coffee drinks, diet soda

While you are in the throes of toxic mold, you already have Chronic Inflammatory Response Syndrome (CIRS).

The last thing you want to do now is choose to eat inflammatory foods. There may be a time that you can tolerate a bit of these foods later, but not right now.

Avoiding processed, microwaveable and pre-made foods helps you avoid inflammatory food chemicals and toxic packaging.

Choose wild-caught, grass-fed organic or organic/small farm/local (even better) to avoid potent pesticides and herbicides.

I'll talk more about avoiding foods that contain mold and special diets for bloating and cellular detox in an upcoming chapter.

Time-Restricted Eating

People are more familiar with the term 'intermittent fasting,' but there is a related practice called time-restricted eating

(TRE) that I think is important because it takes the emphasis off fasting.

As you learn to eat less often, longer fasts may become accessible to you. But what I want to emphasize is:

1. Not snacking
2. Thinking about when you eat, not just what you eat

The body has times it does things best. **Simply changing when you eat and how often can improve your microbiome and your cellular energy.**

My basic TRE maximum is 3-4 times within a 12-hour window. If you are a hypoglycemic snacker or a night owl, it may be harder than you think! Just work up to it slowly.

Once you reach that goal, you can experiment with eating two big, healthy meals, or eating three times within 8-10 hours, etc.

I've been wearing a continuous glucose monitor for the past few weeks and working with a dietician. The results have been fascinating. One thing she asked me to try was moving my carbs to breakfast instead of dinner. Apparently that's when we process them best - little did I know.

Turns out that starch in the morning is WAY better processed than carbs at night. Research studies prove the same; early eaters have a better metabolism and experience more weight loss.

It's also really important to stay hydrated as you experiment with TRE. I have a great interview on intermittent fasting and hydration with Dr. David Jockers and another with Dr. Satchin Panda on circadian rhythm linked in the book resources page, www.toxicmoldguide.com.

Hydrating

You learned about hydration above, so I won't go over it again. Basically, anytime besides mealtimes, have access to filtered water and drink it! Learn more about water filtration options in Part 3 of this book.

ESSENTIAL SUPPLEMENTATION

Before you get fancy with specialized detox supplements, get consistent with basic nutritional supplementation.

Your body needs adequate nutrient levels to function optimally. Modern soil quality and food travel times mean less nutrition in your food. The fresher the food, the more nutritious. Food processing further reduces nutrition and pesticides, herbicides, and food additives make your food literally toxic, giving your detox organs the job of processing and clearing them.

Other external factors like pollution and stress create additional nutrient demands. Nutrients are needed for the thousands of enzymatic processes in your body. They can be used to build hormones and energize cells, or they can be used to clear toxins. **The bigger your detox job, the more nutrients you will need to keep all systems running smoothly.**

The essential supplements I recommend are:

- High-quality multivitamin (with methylated B vitamins)
- Fish oil (triglyceride form and tested for contaminants)
- Magnesium (300 mg magnesium bisglycinate chelate)
- Vitamin D3 with K2 (5,000 IU a day unless getting lots of sun, test yearly)

Extra credit:

- Prebiotic - feeds friendly bacteria, start with lowest dose, I like MegaPre
- Probiotic - take with protein meal, start with lowest dose, I like Megasporebiotic

Here's why these supplements are on my must-have list:

- **High-quality multivitamin** - Depleted soil, stress, and toxins make it tough to get your fill of essential vitamins and nutrients...even if you eat clean. Also, water-soluble vitamins like vitamins B and C can't be stored, so getting them every day is crucial. Taking a daily multivitamin fills in the nutritional gaps to ensure you're getting the essential vitamins and nutrients your body needs.
- **Fish oil** - Omega-3 fatty acids reduce inflammation, a trigger for most chronic illnesses. Research shows fish oil reduces inflammatory cytokines, the very ones that get amped up through mycotoxin exposure. Plus, fish oil is amazing for brain health. In fact, your brain is 60% fat! Fish oil eases depression, supports healthy skin and bones and even aids weight loss.
- **Magnesium** - This mineral is critical for detox, sleep, hormone balance, energy, mood and much more. In fact, magnesium is a cofactor in over 300 enzymatic reactions in your body! That means when you're low on magnesium, *all* those bodily processes suffer. Magnesium helps your body stay in "rest and digest" mode, the state where true healing happens. Stress

depletes magnesium, so it's important to replenish this mineral daily.
- **Vitamin D3 with K2** - Also known as the "sunshine vitamin," Vitamin D is crucial for immunity, hormone support, healthy bones, mood and much more. Nowadays, vitamin D deficiency is rampant, with most people spending the majority of their time indoors. In fact, worldwide, about 50% of people have a vitamin D deficiency! Taking a daily vitamin D supplement ensures you're never low on this vital nutrient, no matter your sunshine status. Combining vitamin D3 with K2 ensures maximum absorption.
- **Prebiotic** - If you suffer from chronic digestive issues, prebiotics can be a gamechanger. These non-digestible fibers feed your friendly bacteria, helping increase microbial diversity. Research shows prebiotics improve your gut barrier, enhance short-chain fatty acid production and even reduce pathogenic bacteria in the gut.
- **Probiotics (preferably spore-based)** - Did you know 70% of your immune system lives in your gut? It's true! Your immunity and overall health depend on a healthy gut. Your gut bacteria support healthy digestion, brain health, and even neurotransmitter production. Probiotics help replenish your stores of these beneficial bacteria. When choosing a probiotic, I *highly* recommend taking a spore-based product. They're designed to withstand the harsh conditions of the gut and arrive in the intestines intact.

Unfortunately many of the supplements for sale in stores are low-quality. They may be affordable, but if they're not absorbable, it's a waste of money. Part of my job as a practitioner is to understand which supplement forms absorb best and provide the best forms to my clients.

Since these essential vitamins are so important to me, I carry the first four in our own Function Detox Products line, and the last two are from our trusted partner. You can find out more at toxicmoldguide.com.

I take my essentials every day about an hour after lunch with water.

SUMMARY

Which of the areas above would you like to focus on? Try not to pick too many at once. For example, start with chewing more and eating slower, plus drinking more water. Once you adjust to those, add something new.

Take-aways:

- Eating correctly is a part of a healthy lifestyle
- Sometimes your values and actions don't match, and you need to course correct
- Smart supplementation starts with the basics, not just fancy extras
- Your best basic diet involves whole foods and plenty of fiber
- Sip filtered water throughout the day between meals
- Prioritize time with yourself, with loved ones and in nature

In the next chapter, I'll dig deeper into diet. I know it can feel SO confusing when deciding what to eat, and right now your digestive system is likely quite sensitive.

Client Story –

Turner had never taken supplements before mold, unless you count taking muscle building powders in high school! Severely affected by mold, he was not thrilled to be spending money on practitioner visits and a grip of supplements that seemed to 'do nothing.'

Following many of the changes in this book, Turner got better and better. He is now in the maintenance stage of healing that you'll learn about in Chapter 13.

Guess what? He now takes his daily essential supplements...by choice! To clarify, he takes our Functional Detox Products magnesium, our multivitamin, CoQ10 (in Chapter 9) and vitamin D. And he tries to eat a high-fiber diet.

As a practitioner, it really makes me smile! He realized over time and with his own trial and error that these things do support him with increased energy, decreased pain and better sleep.

8
MORE ON DIET

IN THIS CHAPTER

- Dietary changes to consider based on certain symptoms
- Why diet is not the only solution
- Why deciding what to eat has become so confusing
- Why fat is not your enemy
- How to eat food

INTRODUCTION

Diet alone is definitely not enough to fix you when you live in a moldy home. And it's not enough when you move out either.

This is a myth I have to bust from time to time. Yes, a good diet is great. You get more nutrition and you feed your friendly bacteria. You avoid inflammatory foods and their effects.

By the time you discover toxic mold illness, you probably have a long list of imbalances in your body. These developed in the somewhat *unnatural* environment of a manufactured home with drywall and indoor plumbing and in the context of stress, WIFI, blue light and man-made chemicals.

So to say, "Well, I'll just eat right and it will get better," is oversimplified and, in my opinion, *impossible* as an approach to heal from toxic mold. I see clients who never detoxed and have a positive urine test for mycotoxins, even though their exposure was years ago.

Nutrition is an accessible subject and *is* important, but it cannot fix multiple gut infections, mold lodged in your brain and sinuses, emotional trauma, congested lymph, etc.

For the record, the other pet peeves of mine on diet are "everything in moderation," and "I get all the nutrients I need from food." These dangerous generalizations do not serve us.

Lastly, saying "there is so much conflicting nutritional information out there that I should just do what I want," does not serve you either. I agree, there is a *ton* of conflicting information. There are diet fads and foods that are touted as both good and bad.

Keep in mind a couple of things:

1. **The best diet for *you* depends on *you* and where *you* are at in your life right now.**

A pregnant woman, a 1-yr old and a very mold-ill menopausal woman will need different diets.

In this chapter, I'll focus on you: the mold-ill person.

2. Nutrition science is evolving.

As humans, we went from survival eating to farming to processed foods and fertilizers, to the modern study of medicine and being able to scientifically test herbs, foods and more. This is exciting stuff! The first vitamin wasn't even discovered until 1913.

This research is valuable for the field of nutrition and developing targeted therapies.

One example is the wealth of information of the microbiome that is under development. We are learning that this bacterial environment in and on our bodies is so critical to our health.

3. **Fads happen.**

The trouble starts when a new dietary 'discovery' is packaged into a slick marketing campaign. An idea with *some* validity got shrink-wrapped into the end-all-be-all.

Going back to point one, the new diet may not be a fit for you. And that's ok. It's up to you to be savvy about these trends. You don't have to try something just because your neighbor loves it. You can look to a trusted health care provider, and do your own research.

Or you can try it, but not get too attached. And maybe keep the parts you liked and toss the parts you didn't. Above all else, don't let these trends stress you out!

In the last chapter I covered a basic good diet. To recap, it's:

- **M**- microbiome-friendly (lots of variety, fiber and omega fatty acids)
- **A**- anti-inflammatory (low in processed foods and sugars)
- **T**- time-restricted (avoiding snacking, conscious of when you eat)
- **H**- hydrating (both through fresh foods and lots of water)

However, there are few more things you might want to keep in mind diet-wise after you do the above. I know that you may have multiple food sensitivities and irregular bowel movements, along with other symptoms like fatigue and skin rashes.

Modifications to your diet can definitely make a difference, just be sure to pair them with other tactics in the next few chapters.

HOW TO EAT

It may seem silly to explain how to eat, but most modern Americans are eating wrong, and this causes digestive symptoms. So before we move into fancy diets, let's get this part right.

This is how not to eat:

- On the go
- Quickly
- Choosing mainly processed foods
- While sucking down a large drink

- While having an argument
- While distracted
- Gulping down air with your food
- Until overly full

This is how to eat:

- Eating mainly whole foods
- Chewing each bite well
- Closing your mouth and breathing through your nose as you chew
- Avoiding drinks at mealtime
- Turning off distractions and eating mindfully
- Eating in the company of friends and loved ones
- On a regular schedule
- Until 80% full

Learning how to eat again can be pretty hard! I am a super fast eater, and I constantly forget to slow down. Try, for a while, counting your chews, or putting your fork down between bites. Take deep breaths (through your nose) and really enjoy your meal.

After your meal, don't rush back to tasks, but instead take a little rest or walk around the block.

We are meant to be in a relaxed state while eating and this supports digestive enzyme production and motility.

Mealtime Supplement Ideas

You may want to consider taking digestive bitters (they usually come in a tincture form) or eating a salad with bitter greens before your meal. I like to take a broad-spectrum digestive enzyme and other people do well with an apple cider vinegar shot or HCl (hydrochloric acid aka stomach acid) with a meal. All these options stimulate general digestion. Supplementing with 500 mg of berberine before a meal can benefit your insulin response to a meal, preventing blood sugar highs and lows.

SPECIAL DIETARY CONSIDERATIONS

Mold in Food

The Great Plains Laboratory did a small study to observe if eating often potentially moldy foods increased urinary mycotoxin levels. According to this study, it did not.

Dr. Shaw, the lab director, speculates that about 98% of the high mycotoxin results they see are from water-damaged buildings.

However, once you are already sick from environmental mold, your body 'encountering' mold in your food could cause a reaction. These foods are often irritating for other reasons too, because they are processed, inflammatory, riddled with pesticides, or are high in histamines (see section 4 of this chapter).

How much are mold toxins in food affecting the general population? It's hard to say. But for you, I think it's best to get to know this list and experiment.

I don't think you need to avoid every item on the list.

For example, I don't eat much dairy, alcohol or corn because these things bother me in different ways. I moderate tea and chocolate because I love these things but too much is a problem for me.

I am careful to buy fresh nuts, toss any that taste rancid, and store them in the fridge or freezer. Please note: Cooking does not kill off the mycotoxins!

15 FOODS THAT GROW MOLD EASILY

- Any grain: whole or in a product like bread or chips
- Grain-fed meat
- Dog food
- Spices, especially red chilli, black pepper, and dry ginger
- Some herbal supplements
- Dairy products
- Cocoa
- Oat, soy or rice milk
- Fruit juice and dried fruit
- Alcohol
- Coffee or tea
- Lunchmeat or salami
- Nuts
- Popcorn
- Leftovers

HOW TO AVOID MOLD IN FOODS

Below are my best ideas for helping you avoid mold in foods, without going crazy!

- Rotate foods in your diet; don't eat the same potentially moldy foods day after day.
- Do not eat foods that give you reactions (but you can retry these foods later).
- Buy organic, high-quality coffee or coffee tested for mycotoxins like Purity or Bulletproof.

- Store nuts, seeds and coffee beans in the fridge or freezer.
- Inspect foods like bread for mold before purchasing.
- Use spices within 3 months.
- Do not eat leftovers beyond a few days.
- Toss any soft fruits that get moldy such as peaches or tomatoes.
- Toss moldy leftovers, jams, soft cheese, hot dogs, lunch meat, yogurt, or peanut butter.
- Use only clean knives and dish rags.
- Do not leave perishable foods out of the fridge for more than 2 hours.
- Do not store an opened can in the fridge: transfer it to a sealed, glass storage container.
- Clean your fridge with 1 Tbs baking soda and a quart of water. Rinse and dry. Do it every 3 months.
- Trim 1 inch past mold on hard cheese or hard vegetables like cabbage or carrot and use a fresh wrap
- When you encounter mold on food, don't sniff it or prod it. Keep it contained and move it to the outside trash can.
- Use a dehumidifier or fan as needed to keep indoor humidity under 40%.
- Buy high-quality herbal supplements.

Chronic Digestive Issues

Your digestive health will likely be disrupted when you've got toxic mold illness. You'll likely have some or all of these symptoms as result:

- Bloating

- Diarrhea
- Constipation
- Abdominal pain
- Multiple food sensitivities
- Nausea
- Excess appetite or lack of appetite

It's also 100% possible to have a disrupted gut and *not* have direct gut symptoms. Skin rashes, mood changes and more are signs of an imbalanced gut.

While you cannot correct the root causes of the above with diet alone, you may need to adjust your diet more radically for a while. Your body may not tolerate 'cheat foods,' and even some healthy foods may not be tolerated.

The reasons for the above symptoms could be:

- **Leaky gut** (increased intestinal permeability)
- **Leaky brain** (increased blood-brain barrier permeability)
- **Candida** or other fungal infection
- **Parasitic infection**
- **Dysbiosis** (imbalance of good and bad bacteria)
- **SIBO** (small intestinal bacterial infection)
- **SIFO** (small intestinal fungal infection)
- *H. pylori* infection
- **Lack of stomach acid** or digestive enzyme production
- **Lack of bile** or bile flow
- **Chronic stress**
- **Deficiency of immune system** and gastrointestinal immune mucosal layer
- **Lack of chewing** (this is an easy one to address!)

- Wrong diet
- Eating disorders

There are probably even more reasons that I'm not recalling at this moment! This is why digestive diagnosis is tricky. We'll dive more into diagnostics later. For now, realize that you could have more than one of the above maladies, causing multiple symptoms.

Go Low FODMAP?

One diet I tried and liked during my own recovery was the low FODMAP diet. **Low FODMAP is mainly used for chronic bloating and SIBO, but my practitioner recommended it to support mitochondrial health.**

FODMAP stands for "fermentable oligo-, di-, mono-saccharides and polyols." These are types of carbohydrates that are resistant to digestion and are mainly broken down by bacteria in your long intestine, producing gas as a potential by-product. Gas, bloating, cramping, constipation or diarrhea could result.

In her book, *Mighty Mito: Power Up Your Mitochondria for Boundless Energy*, Dr. Suzanne Bennett explains that eating high FODMAP foods is a stress on your already stressed digestive system:

> "Eating excessive amounts of fermentable carbohydrates combined with excess bacteria in the gut produces bloating, flatulence, abdominal pain, diarrhea, constipation, and a host of other symptoms leading to inflammation in the body, free radical damage to major organs and mitochondrial dysfunction."

The by-products of a high FODMAP diet can be harmful in the following ways:

1. The gases produced, particularly hydrogen sulfide gas, can inhibit mitochondrial function, already inhibited by toxic mold
2. High production of d-lactic acid causes undue stress on your mitochondria
3. Dysbiosis (bacterial imbalance) can increase
4. IBS (irritable bowel syndrome) can increase
5. LPS (an endotoxin produced by bacteria) can increase

The low FODMAP diet originally seemed very intimidating to me, as many common foods are high FODMAP, including onion, garlic, apples and ripe bananas.

But, in most circumstances, you just eliminate high FODMAPs for 4-6 weeks, and then slowly introduce these foods back, one by one.

There are plenty of delicious low FODMAP foods, including broccoli, almonds and cantaloupe.

While reintroducing foods, I was surprised how much more bloated I became. Some of this may be natural, when you go from low-gas foods to high-gas foods. I was able to bring back most foods, but I know now that grapes, apples and dried food will leave me somewhat gassy and bloated.

This is not to say that *only* high FODMAP foods can upset your stomach. Corn tortillas, raw carrots and dairy items are low FODMAP, but they don't work for my body.

If you suspect or have been diagnosed with SIBO (small intestinal bacterial overgrowth), you may need to stay on a low FODMAP diet for a longer period of time.

To learn more about a low FODMAP diet, see www.toxic-moldguide.com.

Here is a list of high FODMAP foods to be **avoided**:

- **Veggies:** artichokes, asparagus, beetroot, brussel sprouts, cauliflower, garlic, onion, leeks, mushrooms, and snow peas
- **Fruits:** apples, apricots, bananas (ripe), blackberries, cherries, figs, mangoes, nectarines, peaches, pears, plums, and watermelon
- **Grains:** amaranth, barley, rye, and wheat
- **Legumes:** black eyed peas, butter beans, chickpeas, kidney beans, lentils, lima beans, mung beans, and split peas
- **Nuts:** cashews and pistachios
- **Dairy:** cottage cheese, cream cheese, milk, ricotta, and yogurt
- **Sweeteners:** agave nectar, honey, molasses, sorbitol, and xylitol
- **Beverages:** chai tea, chamomile tea, and coconut water

And low FODMAP foods to be **chosen**:

- **Veggies:** bean sprouts, bell pepper, bok choy, carrot, cucumber, eggplant, green beans, kale, lettuce, parsnips, potatoes, spinach, tomato, turnips, and zucchini
- **Fruits:** banana (unripe), blueberries, cantaloupe, grapes, kiwi, lemons, limes, mandarins, oranges, papaya, pineapple, and strawberries

- **Grains:** brown rice, buckwheat, maize, millet, oats, polenta, quinoa, and tapioca
- **Nuts & Seeds:** almonds, macadamia nuts, peanuts, pine nuts, pumpkin seeds, and walnuts
- **Protein:** beef, chicken, eggs, fish, tofu, and tempeh
- **Dairy:** cheddar cheese, cream, feta, lactose-free milk, and parmesan cheese
- **Sweeteners:** beet sugar, maple syrup, rice malt syrup, and stevia
- **Beverages:** almond milk, black tea, coconut milk, coffee, green tea, peppermint tea, rice milk, water, & white tea

Focus on Fats

The high-fat ketogenic diet trended recently and it benefits brain health, as the brain loves fat. But eating a variety of fibers also benefits the brain through the production of short-chain fatty acids.

I like my friend Dr. Anna Cabeca's opinion, shared in her book *Keto Green 16*, that we can move in and out of a state of ketosis (a state of burning fat for fuel), which is probably what our ancestors did. This lets you have more flexibility in your diet.

I do like my clients to emphasize getting more fats, especially if they are new to the concept. One fad diet that was based on 'half-science' was the low-fat craze of the 1980s.

> *"After 1980, the low-fat approach became an overarching ideology, promoted by physicians, the federal government, the food industry, and the popular health media. Many Americans subscribed to the ideology of low fat, even though there was no clear evidence that it prevented heart disease or promoted weight loss. Ironically, in the same decades that the low-fat approach*

> *assumed ideological status, Americans in the aggregate were getting fatter, leading to what many called an obesity epidemic."*
>
> — JOURNAL OF THE HISTORY OF MEDICINE AND ALLIED SCIENCES, VOLUME 63, ISSUE 2, APRIL 2008, PAGES 139–177

Many of my clients, especially women, had it beat into their heads that fat is bad and still avoid it.

We need fats to perform various important functions within the body. Our bodies produce most of the cholesterol we use, but we do get some from our diets. Omega 3 fatty acids are important for brain and gut health, but you also need omega 6 fatty acids, from unprocessed sources, to control inflammation and support your hormones.

Consider:

- Sesame oil (keep in fridge)
- Hemp oil (keep in fridge)
- Fresh-pressed olive oil
- Fresh, raw nuts like walnuts
- Soaked almonds (soak overnight, rinse and eat in morning)
- Chia puddings and porridges
- Wild salmon
- Guacamole
- Sardines
- Paté
- Roast chicken
- Grass-fed butter or ghee

This final section is one that has really piqued my interest lately. Many of the same foods that can contain bothersome mold are also high in histamines (a chemical messenger that triggers inflammation) or are foods that prevent histamines from breaking down.

This histamine issue could be the problem for you more than food-borne mold.

Histamine Intolerance

Histamines are compounds which are released by cells in response to injury and in allergic and inflammatory reactions.

Histamines are broken down in your intestines by the enzyme diamine oxidase (DAO). If you're suffering from poor digestive health, there's a good chance you're running low on DAO. Low DAO eventually causes histamine levels to build up leading to histamine intolerance.

Then histamines from food exposure or other sources build up.

When I interviewed Dr. Jaban Moore, he said that histamines ramp up over time, and then are slow to go back down. This is how it feels in my body.

I find that in the summer months when I'm going to parties and having more alcohol and desserts and dairy (true confessions...forget what you just read), I can handle these dietary transgressions for a while, and then symptoms flare and I have to quit entirely.

Here are some common symptoms of histamine intolerance:

- Headaches or migraines
- Nasal & sinus congestion
- Sneezing
- Fatigue
- Hives or eczema
- Itching
- Flushing
- Digestive issues
- Irregular menstrual cycle
- Nausea or vomiting
- Anxiety
- Racing heart
- Difficulty regulating body temperature
- Dizziness
- Abdominal cramping
- High blood pressure
- Chest tightness

According to Dr. Becky Campbell, author of *The 4-Phase Histamine Reset Plan*, the eight most common causes of histamine intolerance are:

1. Mast Cell Activation Syndrome (MCAS)
2. Gluten intolerance
3. Leaky gut
4. Gut infections
5. Inflammatory digestive disorders
6. Nutrient deficiencies
7. Genetic mutations
8. Certain medications (Aleve, aspirin and Tagamet are common ones)

Other exacerbating factors could be:

- Environmental causes (pollen, dust mites)
- Hormonal excess (estrogen in particular)
- Adrenal dysfunction
- Lack of sleep
- Stress

Mast Cell Activation Syndrome (MCAS)

I cover gut issues a fair amount in this book. If you are experiencing some of the symptoms above and suspect your gut, please do seek treatment.

Mast Cell Activation Syndrome (MCAS), according to Dr. Campbell, is the most likely cause. Mast cells are white blood cells that are triggered during an allergic reaction or other threats. They release histamines and other chemical messengers.

Those 'other threats' include mold, viruses, allergens and environmental toxins. This is where Toxic Mold Illness or CIRS plays right in - your immune system is responding to *so* many threats!

The inflammation that comes with MCAS seems almost inevitable. In fact, it could be the main driver of some of your symptoms.

FOOD DOS AND DON'TS

Diet is key to getting your histamine levels back in check. You'll want to not only avoid histamine-rich foods, but foods that trigger histamine release or block DAO.

The following histamine-rich foods are troublesome for histamine intolerance:

- Alcohol and other fermented beverages
- Fermented foods (yogurt, sauerkraut, vinegar, etc.)
- Cured meats (bacon, sausage, luncheon meats, hot dogs)
- Citrus fruits
- Dried fruit
- Avocadoes
- Eggplant
- Spinach
- Tomatoes
- Aged cheese

There are also several foods that trigger the release of histamine in the body:

- Alcohol
- Bananas
- Chocolate
- Tomatoes
- Nuts (cashew, walnuts, and peanuts in particular)
- Papaya
- Pineapple
- Shellfish
- Strawberry

Plus, some foods block DAO production, which makes it tricky to keep histamines in check. DAO-blocking foods include:

- Alcohol
- Black tea
- Green tea
- Mate tea
- Energy drinks

Besides avoiding these foods and working on the triggers listed above, there are some supplements that can help. These may be especially helpful when you have strong symptoms:

- **DAO enzyme formulas** - help the body break down excess histamine
- **Quercetin** - blocks the release of histamine from mast cells
- **Vitamin C** - needed for DAO production
- **Stinging nettle** - acts as a natural antihistamine
- **Fish oil** - try a higher dose like 3 gm/day
- **Perilla seed extract** - Metagenics has one
- **Claritin** - this has helped me immensely and is non-drowsy
- **Benadryl** - this sleep-inducing antihistamine is sometimes used as a test for MCAS

SUMMARY

- How you eat matters
- Digestive supplements at mealtimes can help
- The best diet for each of us is unique to us, and changes over time
- Histamine intolerance can cause a variety of symptoms
- Many common foods may contain mold
- A low FODMAP diet can relieve bloating, IBS and even help energy
- If you're fat-phobic, think about changing your tune!

In the next chapter, we'll cover one of my very favorite topics - detox techniques.

Client Story –

I'll share my own story here as I've had my ups and downs with diet. As a child, I had ulcers. After living in South America, I developed constipation and probable parasites. In grad school, I developed IBS. And a few years later I moved into a moldy home that brought the IBS back.

Diet is tricky because we are all unique. It's taken me a lot of experimentation and education to find what works best for me- and that project is still not quite complete! I've also had to work on my gut health a lot with rounds of antimicrobials, probiotics and immunoglobulins.

But I can now say that my gut health seems to be quite good. My last stool test looked good, my bowel movements are formed and regular, and I don't have any daily complaints. I still avoid things like gluten, corn products and fried food. I have to keep an eye on my histamine responses to foods. But I've graduated to being able to *occasionally* eat a little decadently!

9
STEP 2: ESTABLISH YOUR DETOX ROUTINE

IN THIS CHAPTER:

- Detox supplements and how to take them
- My favorite and most effective detox techniques
- How to stack detox activities for efficiency

INTRODUCTION

BY NOW YOU'VE learned how to eat right, rest more, get support and get outside. Once your foundations are in place, it's time to start detoxifying.

There are *so* many options for at-home detox. I originally wrote this chapter with a very long list of all the options, but it was overwhelming.

So I decided to present my top five detox supplements and top five detox techniques.

Give these a try, and if you can't tolerate some of them, or you want to stack on more options, I also provide those for you.

In a later chapter I'll provide options to customize your recovery based on the symptoms you are experiencing.

WHY & HOW TO DETOX

Health is a lifestyle, and when your toxic load is high, you need to dedicate to a detox routine.

You can get more and more efficient with your detox lifestyle. Learning anything for the first time takes time, but later it's automatic. **If you are getting side effects or feeling frustrated, go back to Chapter 6 for advice on pacing.**

You can also stack techniques. I'm a big fan of this and so is our friend Connie Zack of Sunlighten Saunas. I'll link my interview with Connie at www.toxicmoldguide.com.

Her idea of stacking is going for a jog or doing yoga before a sauna session. And she's also a fan of light therapy and music while in the sauna.

My idea of stacking is doing a castor oil pack while in the sauna, plus using my red light device, while watching a self-help video (but you don't have to do all this if it's not relaxing!). I'll also do my weekly planner while doing a coffee enema and drinking a green drink or electrolytes.

A weekly planner isn't exactly a healing technique, but it makes the time spent doing a coffee enema more productive.

Our sauna is in the TV room, and I happily watch a show with my son while in the sauna. Again, not directly healing (although comedy can be healing, right?) but it allows me to spend some family time while also detoxing.

Most, but perhaps not all, of these techniques will get you into a relaxed state. We ALL need more of this nowadays! So don't think of it as time wasted, but rather time enjoyed as you shift into a healing parasympathetic state and detox your body.

My Top Detox Supplements:

1. Electrolytes - minimum 1 serving per day, ideally upon waking
2. CoQ10 - 1 serving (200 mg), 1-2 X day
3. Binder - 1 serving 1-3 X day on empty stomach, away from food & medications for 1-2 hours
4. Glutathione - 1 capsule (100 mg) 2 x day with food
5. Broccoli Seed and Sprout - (1-3 day)

My Top Detox Techniques:

1. Sauna - 10-45 minutes - 3-7 X week
2. Coffee enema - as tolerated 1-3 X week
3. Epsom salt bath - 3-7 X week
4. Dry brushing - daily upon waking
5. Mouth taping - nightly

MY TOP SUPPLEMENTS

Electrolytes

Electrolytes are the most tolerated item on this list. Most clean, sugar-free electrolytes will work. I made them a key part of my protocol because:

1. When you have mold illness, you make less antidiuretic hormone (ADH). This means you pee more and potentially lose more electrolytes.
2. Hopefully you are using your sauna (part of this protocol), and you need to restore water and electrolytes lost in sweat.
3. Hydration is an important part of detox, and a clean electrolyte drink will do a great job of hydrating your cells and supporting detoxification.
4. I have found that electrolytes provide me energy, especially when taken first thing in the morning.

How to Take:

Take one serving upon waking as tolerated, during or after sauna, during a work-out, or in a hot temperature. Or just to drink!

I designed my own electrolyte formula, Mi Detox Electrolytes, but other brands I like are Designs for Health and Ultima.

Our supplement has some B vitamins so, if it's too energizing, don't take it in the evening. I find it tolerable on an empty stomach but if you do not, drink it an hour after a meal. Ours is also high in antioxidants to counteract the oxidative effect of toxins.

Electrolytes are generally safe and can be tolerated by children (consider a reduced dose) and in pregnancy or during breastfeeding, but ask your physician if you have any concerns.

You can also make your own electrolytes. There are many variations on the recipe, but here is one for you:

- 12 oz. warm water
- ½ squeezed lemon
- ⅛ tsp Redmond's or Celtic sea salt
- 1 tsp local honey

Mix well and add ice as desired.

CoQ10

Deep fatigue is a hallmark of toxic mold illness. I was so incredibly fatigued that I wanted to sleep forever and never wake up. My brain was also fried; I couldn't hold a thought and had to recall each recent thought at least three times.

These are symptoms of cellular exhaustion. It's a bone-deep fatigue or a complete brain disability. These issues could also appear during hypothyroidism or some other type of poisoning, but any chronic cause of fatigue *causes* cellular fatigue.

What I mean by cellular fatigue is that the mechanism for energy production within the cell is hampered. This condition is more formally called mitochondrial disease and you've probably never heard of it because it's not commonly presented online or in a doctor's office.

If you've got toxic mold illness, your cellular ATP or energy production is being affected by the wandering mycotoxins, able to penetrate your cells, *everywhere*, and able to penetrate the mitochondria of your cells where energy is produced.

CoQ10, also known as Co-enzyme Q10, ubiquinone or ubiquinol, is an antioxidant that your cells produce to counteract the oxidation that occurs when energy is produced.

Energy is produced in a multi-step process that requires many nutrients. While the body does make CoQ10, its production is reduced with age and in the presence of toxins.

This means that right when you need it - when you are low on energy - you are missing a key component of the process.

In addition to supporting energy production and preventing oxidative damage, CoQ10 provides a bounty of benefits, as it supports cellular function in all body systems!

Other benefits:

- Supports cell growth and differentiation
- Supports mitochondrial permeability
- Protects DNA, especially mitochondrial DNA
- Protects lipids and proteins (it's a lipid-soluble antioxidant)
- Recycles vitamin E and C
- Anti-inflammatory
- Benefits 100+ genes
- Supports liver health
- Supports glucose and fat metabolism
- Supports exercise performance and recovery
- Enhances glutathione activity

Dosage: My recommended dosage is 2 soft gels upon waking, equaling 200 mg.

Cautions with CoQ10

CoQ10 should only be taken by those 19 years and older.

CoQ10 and Kidney or Liver Problems

High doses of CoQ10 (300 milligrams or more) may affect liver enzyme levels. Make sure to consult with a trusted healthcare professional.

CoQ10 and Medications

CoQ10 can interact with **blood thinners**, making them less effective in some cases. This includes **warfarin and even aspirin** usage. Make sure to consult with your trusted healthcare professional before supplementing with CoQ10.

Diabetes and hyperglycemia medications: monitor blood sugar levels as your need to medicate may be reduced by CoQ10.

The following medications *reduce* CoQ10 levels, so supplementation with CoQ10 may be especially **helpful**:

- Statins
- Beta-blockers
- Cholesterol medications
- Tricyclic antidepressants

Binders

Binders are the garbagemen of the supplement world - they help make sure the trash (aka toxins) get taken out through the stool.

Binders are substances that 'bind' to toxins to help move them out of the body. Some are highly porous and work by trapping the toxins, others also attract the toxin through a negative charge.

Binders also can bind bile; this is called bile sequestration (which sounds pretty cool to me). Bile will contain toxic compounds, and most bile is recycled to be used again. You can see this issue if you have mycotoxins being excreted through the bile and into the intestines, but then it's just pulled back into the body!

"(Bile acid sequestrants) work by binding negatively charged bile acids and bile salts in the small intestine to interrupt the enterohepatic circulation of bile acids and increase the conversion of cholesterol into bile."

— JOHN R. GUYTON, ANNE CAROL GOLDBERG
IN *CLINICAL LIPIDOLOGY*. 2009

There are many natural binders available, as well as some pharmaceutical options:

- Activated charcoal or bamboo
- Clay
- Chlorella
- Zeolite
- Pectin
- Okra
- Silica
- Fulvic and humic acids
- Cholestyramine (Rx)
- Welchol (Rx)

We have a pair of blogs detailing the qualities of different binders at toxicmoldguide.com.

Dosage: One serving of binders is recommended 1-3 times per day. I normally take one dose at night, but some protocols recommend 3 times per day.

This can get tricky as you need to take them on an empty stomach away from food and other supplements. Some suitable times could be first thing in the morning, last thing at night, or in the middle of the afternoon.

Dr. Neil Nathan explains that you can still be exposed to the toxin even as it is attached to the binder *as it is loosely bound to the binder*, so *sensitive patients may feel worse from taking binders.*

Only take as much binder as you can handle without side effects, *even if it's just a 1/4 capsule every other day, or none at all.*

Most binders should be taken 1 hour before or 2 hours after food and medication.

Most binders are not meant for on-going daily use, as they can prevent optimal nutrient absorption. A particularly strong binder in this regard is charcoal, whereas pectin is much gentler.

One solution to over-binding is 'binder rotation,' in which you simply take a pectin for a while, and then a zeolite, etc.

When I developed our brand, Mi Toxin Binder, I originally left out charcoal in favor of gentler binders. But I just didn't feel it worked as well. Just know that a strong binder is not meant for prolonged use, but instead more cyclic use. So perhaps it's 2 months on, 1 off. Or 5 days on, 2 off. And avoid mealtimes.

I notice that clients can get a little overly preoccupied with taking binders. **As long as you are pooping, sweating and peeing every day, and not experiencing side effects from your detox protocol, you don't always need a binder.**

Binders can also be constipating, which will inhibit good detoxification. So if your binder is causing this, decrease the dosage or add a bowel mover like magnesium citrate.

Mi Toxin Binder includes aloe vera powder and Chinese rhubarb to help keep your bowels moving.

One last note: binders do not do a complete job of binding, so I don't want you to be too nervous that they are sponging up every good thing you've ever eaten!

I learned this from experience; when I've taken a binder and then couldn't fall asleep so I took a melatonin supplement. The melatonin still did the job - it didn't get swallowed up by the binder!

Glutathione

Glutathione is called the master antioxidant of the body. It is very much needed for detoxification, but will become depleted when the toxic load is too high.

This is especially true for mold illness, as mycotoxins decrease the gene expression of the enzymes needed to produce glutathione. This is why several animal studies link mycotoxins exposure with reduced glutathione levels.

That's bad news, as glutathione helps your body in many ways:

- Combats free radical damage

- Supports phase 1 and 2 detox
- Reduces risk of cancer
- Regulates cell apoptosis (cell death)
- Boosts energy production (ATP)
- Acts as a cofactor for several enzymes
- Improves insulin sensitivity
- Regulates gene expression
- Helps your body regenerate vitamin C and E
- Supports immune health

Like many nutrients, glutathione has an active and inactive state. The inactive state is called oxidized glutathione (GSSG) and the active form is called reduced glutathione (GSG). Your body recycles glutathione from its oxidized state (GSSG) into the active form (GSG).

As I mentioned before, glutathione can also be produced by the body. This requires the amino acids cysteine, glutamic acid, and glycine, which are the precursors to glutathione production.

N-acetyl-cysteine (NAC), the precursor to the cysteine, is often taken to bump up glutathione levels. Hospitals have even used N-acetyl-cysteine (NAC) as treatment for poisoning for this very reason!

Your body can recycle glutathione, or make it. It is found in foods like cruciferous veggies and can be taken as a supplement. It also increases with coffee enema use, covered in my top five techniques.

Does Glutathione Cause Side Effects?

When using glutathione as a supplement, you may find you feel better, worse or neutral!

Side effects are rare, but could include:

- Abdominal pain
- Bloating
- Skin rashes
- Breathing problems.

Glutathione for me, like binders, doesn't really feel like much. But I know they are doing good things for me so I take them.

But I've had clients feel instantly better or worse on a binder or on glutathione. If you feel worse, reduce the dosage. If it's still a problem, take a break from it and try it again when you're feeling stronger (i.e. have made progress in your recovery).

Forms of Glutathione - Which is Best?

There are several forms of supplemental glutathione. We carry one by Results RNA that is a micro-ionized spray. This is a good option for kids and people who need dosing options.

There are also liposomal glutathione formulas that usually come in a liquid form. These are very well-absorbed and good for those who can't swallow pills or need dosing options.

I am also a huge fan of S-acetyl-glutathione. This type of glutathione is formulated in a way that prevents it from breaking down in the gut, enhancing absorption. It has an acetyl group attached to the sulfur atom of cysteine in the glutathione molecule which protects the glutathione from breaking down in the gastrointestinal tract. Once absorbed and inside the cells, the acetyl group is removed, leaving the glutathione molecule intact.

We carry a Glutathione Synergy product that contains this highly-absorbable form, along with NAC and B6, which also boost glutathione production.

N-acetyl cysteine (NAC) is a precursor of L-cysteine; glutathione is primarily made up of three amino acids: glutamine, glycine and cysteine. For some people, NAC is better tolerated than glutathione, and it can be more affordable. I prefer to include 'straight' glutathione as well though.

When it comes to glutathione supplementation, you get what you pay for. Many glutathione supplements are poorly absorbed and a waste of money. Be sure you do your homework and choose one of the forms mentioned above so you get the most bang for your buck.

Per daily serving, our Glutathione Synergy contains:

- 1 gm NAC
- 200 mg s-acetyl glutathione
- 10 mg B6

Broccoli Sprout and Seed

No detox protocol is complete without a mention of broccoli sprouts. Broccoli sprouts' detox powers come from the compound sulforaphane, a sulfur-rich compound found in cruciferous veggies like cauliflower, cabbage, bok choy, kale, arugula, collards, watercress, and yes...broccoli!

Eating more cruciferous vegetables will up your sulforaphane alone. But broccoli sprouts amp the effects *way* up. In fact, broccoli sprouts have 100 times the sulforaphane as regular broccoli!

That's why we carry Broccoli Sprout and Seed in our shop. Thanks to its sky-high sulforaphane content, its detox powers are unmatched - *especially* when it comes to mycotoxin detox. And it's way more convenient than chomping down pounds of broccoli every day!

How Sulforaphane Supports Mycotoxin Detox

For starters, sulforaphane activates the NrF2 pathway, supporting phase 1 liver detox. The Nrf2 pathway, known as the "master redox switch," activates your DNA to produce more antioxidants, *including* glutathione. In fact, research shows sulforaphane has more potent effects on Nrf2 than milk thistle, curcumin, and resveratrol!

The sulforaphane in broccoli sprouts supports phase 2 liver detox as well, especially the glucuronidation pathway. This pathway is particularly important for mold illness, as glucuronidation helps remove mycotoxins.

Glucuronidation also helps your body detox excess estrogen, which is especially helpful if you're prone to estrogen dominance.

Other foods and nutrients that support glucuronidation:

- All cruciferous veggies (broccoli of course, but especially broccoli sprouts)
- Citrus fruits
- Dandelion
- Rosemary
- Resveratrol
- Curcumin
- Rooibos tea
- Astaxanthin

While I typically tell our mold patients to take our Broccoli Sprout & Seed to aid mycotoxin detox, its liver-protecting effects support chemical detox as well. Win win!

Dosage: 1 per day for maintenance, 3 per day for acute detox as tolerated

Caution: While broccoli sprouts offer a ton of benefits, if you're on medication you'll need to be cautious, as glucuronidation metabolizes medications as well. As always, talk with your doctor first.

MY TOP TECHNIQUES

Sauna

Sauna increases body temperature, which encourages detoxification. It also:

- Mobilizes toxins of all types; chemicals, mycotoxins, and heavy metals
- Improves immune function
- Lowers inflammation
- Helps repair and regenerate cells
- Turns off sympathetic dominance (stress mode) and turns on relaxation state
- Activates mitochondrial activity & ATP production
- Activates heat shock proteins to repair cellular damage
- Can aid in weight loss
- Assists in detoxification (especially far infrared)
- Increases BDNF, brain-derived neurotrophic factor
- Improves sleep quality

It has *so* many benefits that it is a 'required' part of my mold protocol with clients.

Getting Started

Set a time limit in the very beginning. Your body will not be able to tolerate an hour-long session at first.

Take it slow with ten to fifteen minute sessions until you are able to sit in your sauna and sweat it out for a half hour or more. Listen to your body--if your body says it's time to get out, just get out!

For kids, a rule of thumb is one minute of sauna time x their age. But I find that many kids can tolerate more than that, especially if the temperature is slower and/or their head and upper body can remain out of the sauna.

Session lengths and temperatures can vary. What's most important is to do what you tolerate. That may start with 10 minutes at a lower temperature. That may also be all that children can tolerate. Now I usually do about 40 minutes at a high heat of 140 degrees.

Make sure that you are drinking enough water to remain hydrated with your treatments.

Never skip the shower after a sauna! You need to rinse off topical toxins. Use soap and shampoo your hair.

I tolerate sauna usage very well and it gave me immediate relief when I was at my sickest. But some of my clients can only tolerate short, infrequent or not-so-hot sessions because they can't handle that level of detoxification. As always, do what is a fit for your body at this point.

According to Connie Zack, co-owner of Sunlighten Saunas, *frequency* is what's most important. She likes a minimum of three times a week and I agree. You can do it daily, as long as you are staying well-hydrated and nourished and feel fine.

Deluxe Detox Routine

These are not required, but you may want to experiment with them:

1. **Use glutathione before getting in the sauna.** This can be 100 mg of a liquid or capsule, or 12 sprays of our ACG glutathione.
2. **Drink electrolytes.** You can do this during or after your sauna. Try our Mi Detox Electrolytes, make a DIY batch, or you can drink coconut water.

3. **Take binders.** To make sure toxins continue outward and don't recirculate back into you, take 2 capsules of our Mi Toxin Binder or another binder after your sauna and away from food and medications.
4. **Bathe with charcoal soap after the sauna.** The above binding supplement contains charcoal. Charcoal can also be used in toothpastes, masks, or in a soap! Check out the charcoal bar soap from Beautycounter as a way to really pull those toxins off of you after a sauna.

Choosing a Sauna

What is most important is that you get started with sweating. If you are displaced due to mold, using a sauna at an affordable gym or club is a great starting point.

With COVID, this may be less available. So the second option I'll present is an affordable, portable sauna or sauna blanket. You can buy this for a temporary living situation or a small space. Be careful not to let your sauna get contaminated by a moldy environment.

A sauna blanket is a charged blanket that wraps around you like a sleeping bag. I've heard good things about the brand Higher Dose.

The next level is a more permanent fixture sauna. Do not buy this unless you are now in a mold-free environment!

Besides considering your budget and your space, consider these factors:

- Reliability of brand
- Off-gassing
- EMF levels
- Type of heat

I now own a Sunlighten Solo System which is a more mobile, one-person sauna, but it's also very sturdy and will last many years. It doesn't require special wiring and doesn't take up a ton of space.

My Solo System is a far infrared wavelength only. This wavelength is best for detoxification. Near and mid-range infrared also have benefits and are available in other saunas, including cabin saunas by Sunlighten. You can call Sunlighten to find the best match for you and mention me and ask for any current specials.

Dry Brushing

A dry brush is a natural bristle brush to brush your dry skin to move lymph and blood.

When your body is overloaded with toxins, the lymph - the fluid that takes out the trash - can get backed up. You may notice puffy eyes, ankle edema or a congested feeling in the groin creases.

Dry brushing also increases circulation to your skin, leaving you feeling invigorated and more 'awake' and ready for the day. Lastly, it can help prevent cellulite and exfoliate your skin, so it's a beauty treatment too.

How to Get Started

When your skin is dry, brush from your extremities towards your heart (not back and forth) using a long stroke that is firm but not deep. Brush over an area at least a few times. For small areas like palms, you can opt for a circular motion. You can also use a smaller brush for areas like the face and neck.

You can do a longer session of dry brushing and hit every area, but you can also do a quicker version and just hit all the large surface areas.

If you have a brush with a handle, it's easier to reach your back. I like to pay special attention to my groin crease and armpit area as these areas collect lymph. These areas may do better with a smaller brush as well.

You may need to use a softer brush or a lighter stroke when you are just getting used to it. You can shower after brushing, but you don't need to do so.

A good brush or brush set costs $10-$35. We currently offer one in our shop, accessible through toxicmoldguide.com.

Coffee Enema

Enemas themselves date back hundreds of thousands of years. Hippocrates touted their benefits and some scholars have suggested that enemas were detailed as a form of bodily purification and cleansing in the dead sea scrolls. Enemas apply a medicinal liquid into the lower bowel via the rectum.

Coffee contains certain compounds, *kahweol palmitate* and *cafestol palmitate*, both of which can increase glutathione production. Glutathione is essential for optimal detoxification and mitigating free radical damage.

Coffee also contains a compound called theophylline, which can help to reduce inflammation in both the intestines and liver.

Caution: coffee enemas are not a fit for everyone! If you have mobility issues (such as getting on and off the floor), gallbladder issues, hemorrhoids or anal fissures, abdominal cramping or extreme caffeine sensitivity, they may not be a bit for you. *Please discuss it with your doctor before trying it.*

I got so much more energy quickly when I was really sick and exhausted that I felt I had to include coffee enema in my top four. It was honestly a game changer for me.

You'll need:

- Light roast organic coffee (must be caffeinated)
- Filtered water
- Gloves
- Enema kit

Boil 2.5 cups of water. Add 4 Tbs coarse ground coffee. Wait 15 minutes. Add 2 cups of room temperature water. Strain out coffee grounds.

(Recipe shared with permission of Dr. Jay Davidson from his book, *Five Steps to Restoring Health Protocol: Helping Those Who Haven't Been Helped with Lyme Disease, Thyroid Problems, Adrenal Fatigue, Heavy Metal Toxicity, Digestive Issues, and More.*)

Add brewed coffee to a sealed enema bag (valve closed). Now open the valve to release air in the hose and let the coffee come to the bottom of the hose.

Set up in a bathtub on or a bathroom floor with comfy towels and a pillow. Your coffee enema kit will have an insertion tip at the end of the hose.

Put on your gloves and place the insertion tip about 2-3 inches into your rectum. You can use coconut oil or glycerin as a lubricant if you want.

Open the valve and SLOWLY allow the coffee to flow. If your bag is hanging too high, the flow may be too fast. I like the bag just a couple feet higher than me.

I usually do 3 rounds. The fist is just a warm-up and I don't add a lot of coffee nor retain it for a long time (maybe 5 minutes). You will have more of an urge to have a bowel movement on the first round. Some people use plain warm water on the first round.

For the second round, I can put in more coffee and retain it for longer, maybe 10 minutes. But if I add too much coffee too quickly I won't be able to retain the coffee and I'll need to use the toilet.

The mistake most people make is to release coffee too quickly. That is hard to retain. It's better to add little by little.

By the third round, my body is used to it and I can hold more coffee for a longer time. It's no problem to hold it for 15-20 minutes.

Sometimes I do a fourth round if I have more coffee. Supposedly you can hold 2 cups at once, but I often can't, so I just go with that and do more rounds if I want.

It will take you at least a few tries to get comfortable with doing coffee enemas. **If you have issues with: gallbladder congestion, anal fissures, hemorrhoids, immobility, etc., they may** not be a fit for you! Please ask your supervising physician if you are unsure.

If you are coffee or caffeine sensitive, you may feel too much a kick from an enema, but you may not. I am caffeine sensitive and I still do them.

I use a bag enema kit by Aussie Health Co. I normally use coffee I buy locally, but you can also use Purity, Bulletproof, Life Boost or another high-quality online brand. Cost is around $20-40 to get started.

Epsom Salt Baths

Epsom salt baths are so easy and enjoyable that it's more like a treat than actual work. But they *do* have real benefits! You can add essential oils or other beneficial ingredients to your bath as well.

Epsom salt is also known as magnesium sulfate - a chemical compound made up of magnesium, sulfur, and oxygen that absorbs through your skin.

Epsom salts contain both sulfur and magnesium that support detoxification. Soaking in a bath is a way to get these nutrients if you can't take pills, plus you are getting direct muscle relaxation.

Epsom salt baths can help calm the nervous system, relax cramps, reduce pain and swelling, promote sleep and healthy bowel movements.

How do I do it?

The basic practice is adding 2 cups of Epsom salts into a tub of warm running water. But you can also add in a few drops of essential oil to deepen your experience. I like basil for muscle pain, lavender for relaxation, ylang ylang for relaxation and clary sage for hormonal complaints.

Another technique is to use 1 cup of Epsom salt paired with 1/2 cup of baking soda. This is also supposed to help clear the harmful effects of EMF.

While there may not be scientific evidence to back this up, baking soda and Epsom salts are purported to help you recover from EMF exposure from electronic devices, cell service and Wi-Fi.

I have also used them for panic attacks and energetic clearing. They are a great way to release the influences felt during a long day, or calm yourself in an emotional crisis.

A bag of Epsom salt is about $5-$10 and can be purchased at Costco, health food stores and most drugstores.

Mouth Taping

Mouth taping is literally taping your mouth shut at night with a piece of bandage tape placed horizontally across your mouth.

What's the benefit?

We are meant to breathe through our noses, not our mouths, but sometimes we sleep with mouths wide open. It's estimated that between 30-50% of adults are mouth breathers. Mouth taping can return you to the benefits of nose breathing:

- Improved oral health (including breath odor, plaque and cavities)
- Improved sleep
- Increased immunity
- Decreased inflammation & allergies
- Better mood

Nasal breathing encourages nitric oxide production, an important signaling molecule for energy and blood flow.

How do I do it?

It's about the easiest thing to do - simply tape your mouth shut! Use a gentle bandage tape, but I've used scotch tape in a pinch just fine. There is a brand called SomniFix that sells boxes of strips that are really nice. If you tend to have nasal congestion, use a nasal wash or a silver nasal spray beforehand so your nasal passages are clear. If you can't breathe through your nose, don't tape your mouth shut!

I actually recommend the nasal spray regardless - it will moisten and detoxify your nose for your sleeping hours. You can use lip balm before applying the tape to protect your lips. Simply peel off the tape in the morning.

I was a major mouth breather and I'd wake up with a sore throat *often*, especially in the winter. This would give me malaise and aches that would sometimes take half a day to kick, and then it might start all over the next day. Mouth taping was a game changer for my health! Tape cost is $5-20.

SUMMARY

- There's a lot you can do at-home to detox!
- Everyone responds differently; cater your routine
- You can save time by detox stacking

In the next chapter, we'll take a deeper dive into a more customized and recovery plan based on your unique symptoms.

My Story -

I was wary of coffee enemas, but I learned more about the procedure from Dr. Jay Davidson while reading his book, mentioned above.

Soon after, I interviewed him on my podcast, and I was still fairly sick from mold at the time. I asked him, 'Should I really do this?' And he said it's been a big help to many people, so I decided to take the plunge.

They were a huge relief to me when I was at my sickest- lifting me out of lethargy for at least half a day. Many clients come to me *already* established coffee enema fans as well.

I am now a huge fan of coffee enemas and people now often ask *me* about them when I get interviewed! I still do a coffee enema about once a week.

10
MORE DETOX TECHNIQUES

IN THIS CHAPTER

- Benefits, costs and how to on more detox techniques

INTRODUCTION

SOME OF THESE techniques cost money, and others are free. Some require practitioners, others do not. **Don't be fooled into thinking that more expensive/more exotic equals more effective!** That's not always the case.

Sometimes the hero just calmly cooks bone broth, takes an Epsom salt bath, meditates and goes to bed early. She didn't spend a lot of money or travel to see a specialist, but she's getting better, bit by bit.

Remember that the emotional centers and other areas of your brain can be affected by mold. And that your cells will best heal when you are in a relaxed state.

Also you need free-flowing blood and lymph to best heal, from simple things like exercise, massage and stretching. **So don't disregard the importance of just taking good care of your physical and mental health!**

DETOX TECHNIQUES A-Z

Acupuncture

What is it?

Acupuncture is a part of traditional Chinese medicine in which fine, sterile needles are inserted along energy pathways to affect organ function, ease pain and stimulate a parasympathetic state.

What's the benefit?

Acupuncture can help for lots of things that concern the mold client: pain, headaches, poor digestion, insomnia and more. It can be a nice option if supplement sensitive or if chronically stressed. It gently supports a body that's been depleted by toxicity.

How do I do it?

Acupuncture must be performed by a licensed practitioner, and usually multiple sessions are required. Your acupuncturist may also recommend herbs or perform other therapeutic modalities.

What's the cost?

Costs can range from $200 to $25. Your insurance may cover acupuncture, or you may utilize a community clinic or 'chain' clinic that offers drop-in service and a lower cost.

Castor Oil Packs

What is it?

Castor oil packs are a castor-oil soaked cloth that you wrap or apply to the body, usually at the abdomen.

What's the benefit?

Castor oil is high in antioxidants and encourages glutathione recycling. It can relieve constipation or IBS while decreasing gut inflammation and supporting nutrient absorption. It can be used for menstrual complaints. Castor oil can also be used to regrow hair, cleanse the skin and support restful sleep.

Castor oil packs almost made my top 5 picks, by the way!

How do I do it?

Castor oil packs are applied externally with a flannel or similar material. They are placed over the abdomen, liver, kidneys, uterus, or the lungs occasionally. A pack is retained for 30 minutes overnight.

I love the brand Queen of Thrones that offers a modern style castor oil pack that is much less messy than traditional flannel packs. They also offer organic castor oil in a glass bottle. I linked it in the appendix, along with an interview with the company's founder and a quick instructional video.

What's the cost?

$20-$60 (lasts a long time)

Chiropractic Medicine

What is it?

Chiropractic medicine involves manual manipulation of the spine and other joints of the body. When the spine is in proper alignment the central nervous system can work more effectively, enhancing the body's natural ability to heal.

What's the benefit?

Chiropractic medicine is used to improve joint mobility, ease back and neck pain, and decrease headaches. It can also be done preventatively to keep the body in proper alignment.

How do I do it?

Chiropractic medicine is done by a licensed chiropractor. Each session involves a spinal adjustment, but may also include stretching, spinal traction, transcutaneous electric nerve stimulation (TENS), or nutritional counseling.

What's the cost?

On average, each chiropractic treatment costs about $65, but treatments range from $35-$100 depending on your practitioner. Check with your insurance, as they may cover some of the cost.

Cryotherapy

What is it?

Cryotherapy is using a very cold room or chamber (-200 to -300 degrees F) for therapeutic benefits. There are also cryotherapy wands that can be applied to local areas or pain or aesthetics.

What's the benefit?

Cryotherapy can remote immune adaptability and exercise recovery. The cold temperature is anti-inflammatory. It also burns a high number of calories to be in the chamber. It can improve mood and cognition. https://www.healthline.com/health/cryotherapy-benefits#

How do I do it?

There are cryotherapy centers that may also offer sauna, red light therapy, IV therapy, etc. I love that these different chains are popping up! The local one I like is US Cryotherapy. I got a very affordable 10-pack of visits and I get 3 modalities each time I visit.

Be sure to work with a trained professional so you don't over-expose yourself.

What's the cost?

$30-$65. Sessions are often sold in packages to bring the price down. You may be able to find a Groupon to try it. Chambers can be purchased or leased for at-home use as well.

Essential Oils

What is it?

Essential oils are the aromatic compounds of plants, roots and flowers.

What's the benefit?

Essential oils are high in antioxidants and contain compounds that have positive effects on the body. They can calm the nervous system, increase hormone production, fight infections and more.

How do I do it?

Essential oils are generally either applied topically with a carrier oil or inhaled. The topic is quite broad so I'll provide some links in the appendix to learn more.

Just before I got really sick, I purchased about 15 essential oil blends. When I had *so* many different daily symptoms, essential oils were a wonderful, pill-free way to manage some of these.

While essential oils *can* address mold directly, I think they are best considered for the array of symptoms they can support. Here are a few ideas:

- Headaches and fatigue - peppermint
- Lymph congestion in neck or groin - citrus oils like orange, lemon or grapefruit
- Stress and panic - lavender

Some oils are 'hot' and should not be applied directly to the skin. Oil dilution is more of a concern when treating children. I 100% recommend essential oils and think every family should have a collection, but learn first and proceed with caution.

I recommend the essential oil books by Dr. Mariza Snyder, Dr. Eric Zielinski and Jodi Cohen.

What's the cost?

$10-$50 per oil

Green Drink

What is it?

This is a simple light drink with greens and lemon as the dominant ingredients.

What's the benefit?

Green drinks are hydrating, alkalizing and contain nutrients that support red blood cells, the liver and general detoxification.

When I was getting some treatment while still quite sick, a chiropractor told me my blood was dark and sticky. This didn't sound good.

I looked into blood detoxifiers and started to take chlorella and make this drink. I definitely felt more energized from the practice.

How do I do it?

Here's the recipe:

Cilantro Lime Drink Recipe

- 12 oz. of purified, cool water to your blender
- 1 squeezed lime or small lemon
- 1 generous handful of organic, washed broccoli sprouts, spinach or other green
- 1 medium handful of organic, washed cilantro
- 1 teaspoon of local honey
- Blend thoroughly
- Strain, pour and drink within 15 minutes

What's the cost?

About $1 a serving

Hyperbaric Oxygen Therapy (HBOT)

What is it?

Hyperbaric oxygen therapy (HBOT) is a treatment that utilizes greater than normal atmospheric pressure, sometimes in combination with 100% oxygen. A session in a hyperbaric oxygen chamber is usually an hour and may involve an extra oxygen mask for your nose and mouth.

What's the benefit?

Data has shown that chronic mold exposure can result in impaired brain function.

Evidence from one study supports the use of HBOT as a mold toxicity treatment. At a relatively low pressure of 1.3 ATA, patients suffering from mold exposure experienced significant relief. Patients received 10 treatments that lasted approximately 90 minutes each. **At the end of the study, researchers concluded patients improved their attention span, reaction time, and consistency.**

HBOT also has a calming effect on the nervous system that is a welcome relief from the chronic stress of mold illness.

HBOT has also been used for Lyme disease as oxygenating the tiniest capillaries where infection hides is a novel approach. I suspect, in my case, it is also effective for Epstein Barr virus.

How do I do it?

Sessions in an HBOT last 60-90 minutes and it's usually recommended to do 30 sessions when brain injury is involved. The bulk of study on HBOT has been on traumatic brain injury and post-traumatic stress disorder.

Know that when you are using HBOT for infection you may have a die-off reaction. This unexpectedly happened to me. Start with HBOT just once a week at first and increase to twice a week as tolerated.

What's the cost?

$50 - $10,000. I bought a small package of reduced price sessions on Groupon. Later I bought a used at-home chamber on Craig's List.

You can certainly utilize a therapy center, but prepare to do at least 10-30 sessions. I decided to buy a unit so I could be more time-efficient, and I can always sell it later to recoup some of my investment.

Holistic Dental Care

What is it?

Holistic dentistry is an alternative form of dental care that believes in the mouth-body connection, which is the idea that your oral health and whole body health are related.

What's the benefit?

Holistic dental care's main benefit is avoiding toxins. Holistic dentists avoid toxic materials like mercury and fluoride. Instead, they opt for natural, biocompatible materials like porcelain, ceramic, and resin. Biocompatible means the materials work well on the whole body and are not known for causing allergic reactions, which is especially helpful if you're in the midst of mold recovery.

Another benefit is that holistic dentists understand that the health of the mouth can mimic the patient's overall health. Rather than strictly focusing on the mouth, they may make nutritional, sleep, or breathing recommendations that improve whole body health.

How do I do it?

Book a consultation with a holistic dentist in your area. Because the focus is whole-body, they'll gather a thorough health history and additional information that could be impacting your health like lifestyle, stress, nutrition, and sleep habits.

If you're having trouble finding a holistic dentist in your area, I've listed a helpful resource in the appendix.

You can also try some DIY holistic dental care simply by swapping out your dental products for more natural ones.

What's the cost?

Because they use safer materials and less invasive treatments, holistic dental care does cost more on average than traditional dental care. Contact your holistic dentist for pricing.

IV Therapy

What is it?

IV therapy, also called infusion therapy is a method of delivering fluids, nutrients, or medications directly into the bloodstream. It can include IV glutathione, NAD, vitamin C and more.

What's the benefit?

The main benefit of IV vitamin therapy is it increases cellular absorption of nutrients. Getting nutrients via an IV allows them to bypass the digestive system and be more readily absorbed. This can be especially helpful for people with chronic digestive issues who may eat well and take supplements, but struggle with absorption.

Additional benefits will vary depending on what ingredients are in your nutrient cocktail. Some of the most common are:

- Enhanced immunity
- Increased energy
- Detoxification support
- Restoration of depleted vitamin and mineral levels
- Rehydration

How do I do it?

IV therapy is performed by a nurse or other health practitioner. An average session lasts about 30 minutes to an hour and effects can last up to a few days after your session.

What's the cost?

$125-$200 depending on your unique IV formula

Lymphatic Massage

What is it?

Lymphatic drainage massage is a very gentle, superficial massage with a qualified professional to boost lymphatic movement and drainage.

What's the benefit?

Lymphatic massage can reduce swelling and inflammation and promote detoxification.

How do I do it?

Lymphatic massage is not as popular as Swedish and deep tissue massage, but it's very relaxing and is specially designed to move lymph. It's more popular with those who have had surgery but it works great for mold too.

The first time I went I dumped a lot of toxins and hadn't taken binders so I felt poorly afterwards. But it passed quickly and subsequent sessions were just fine.

It's usually best to do a series of treatments.

What's the cost?

$60-$150 per session

Massage

What is it?

Massage is the practice of manipulating the soft tissues of the body in order to relieve pain and induce relaxation.

What's the benefit?

Massage has a *ton* of health benefits including:

- Easing muscle tension
- Relieving stress
- Improving circulation
- Reducing pain
- Improving sleep
- Relieves headaches
- Enhances immunity
- Promoting relaxation response
- Easing symptoms of depression
- Reducing anxiety

How do I do it?

Be sure you know your massage goals before booking an appointment. While there are a ton of massage varieties, the two mainstays are Swedish and deep tissue. Swedish massage promotes relaxation with gentle, long strokes and circular motions. Deep tissue massage uses slower, more intense strokes to target deep layers of muscle tension.

There are a lot of massage subscription clubs nowadays that make getting regular massage more affordable. But you can always go the free route and incorporate some DIY massage into your weekly routine. Inject some self love in your yoga or stretching practices by ending with a foot rub. Or you can recruit a family member to swap shoulder and neck massages.

What's the cost?

Professional massages run around $85-$125 a session.

Meditation

What is it?

Meditation comes in a handful of different forms, but it's essentially calming and observing the mind and/or the breath to achieve a more peaceful state.

What's the benefit?

Meditation can yield many benefits: better sleep, increased patience and kindness, more frequent contentment, clearer thinking and decision making, and even a longer lifespan!

How do I do it?

The biggest barrier to entry with mediation usually comes from expecting too much too soon. It may seem boring, like nothing is happening, or you aren't doing it right, or you'd be better off doing about *anything* other than this.

It is completely out of our cultural norm to 'do nothing' and to observe the mind and breath. But, if you start doing it regularly, and learning a bit about it, you will likely find it helpful.

My favorite type of meditation is timed mindfulness meditation. Using a timer, even if it's only for 3 minutes, creates a frame for your meditation.

Mindfulness meditation reignites your observation of the present moment. You can look out a window, sit outside, or sit quietly in bed. Observe what you see, any sounds, air movement. Notice your body and breath. Are you tight? Is your jaw clenched? Let that unwind and relax into your space.

When I was at my sickest, I did 10 minutes of timed mindfulness meditation per day. I think it really helped me stay grounded in the midst of a chaotic time. Remember that healing happens in a relaxed parasympathetic state. How often are you in that state??

Lately, I aim for twice a day, and I do a mix of timed meditation and guided meditation. I use the app Insight Timer. It's totally free but you can donate to teachers or purchase a course.

What's the cost?

It's free! But you may want to take a class, join a group or read a book about it. You can also download Insight Timer from your phone's app store.

Nasal Rinse

What is it?

Nasal rinsing is performed with a Neti pot or squirt or spray bottle with the goal of rinsing debris and mucus out of the nose.

What's the benefit?

Allergens, dust and mold spores can lodge in the mucous membranes of the nose, as well as the sinus cavities. This physical modality can remove irritants and take stress off the immune system.

There is also a mold-related infection you can get in your nose called MARCoNS. MARCoNS stands for Multiple Antibiotic Resistant Coagulase Negative Staphylococci. The presence of this infection in your nose can weaken your immune system and decrease the production of melatonin, an important hormone and antioxidant for sleep and immunity.

This is something you can test for, and/or you can do the protocol below.

How do I do it?

You may be familiar with Neti pots - small pots with a spout and you tilt your head to allow saline water into your nostril.

I prefer a couple of other options:

1. NeilMed Sinus Rinse - this comes with its own gentle saline packets and it's super easy to use. Use with distilled or filtered water. I did this twice daily for over a year when I was quite mold ill.
2. ACS silver nasal spray - if you're not dealing with a major sinus or mold problem, using this quick spray and both moisturizes your nasal cavity, cleans out irritants and helps kill germs. I use this every morning and a little extra if traveling.

If you want to address MARCoNs or other possible infections in the nose, including mold infections, you can try the following protocol:

Add 10 drops Biocidin tincture or Biocidin LS to one bottle ACS Silver Spray. Spray 2 sprays in each nostril 3 times a day for 2 months.

Please note that MARCoNs infections can be super stubborn. In current practice, many practitioners treat this last or not at all, feeling it's not the dominant issue in an array of issues.

I've got a supportive article about nasal washing and links to the above items in the appendix.

What's the cost?

$10-$20

Oil Pulling

What is it?

Oil pulling is swishing and gargling oil and pulling it though your teeth.

What's the benefit?

Oil pulling offers many benefits, including: breaking up biofilms (including plaque), preventing infections in your mouth from traveling to your gut, preventing bad breath and gum disease, reducing inflammation, improving the oral microbiome.

You can harbor infections and bacterial overgrowth in the mouth that can really stress the body. Practicing 'super care' of your mouth with habits like oil pulling, water picking and chewing xylitol gum can help.

How do I do it?

Simply put a spoonful of oil (I use coconut) into your mouth and swish and pull it through the cracks in your teeth. You can also use sesame, sunflower or olive oil.

You can oil pull up to 15-20 minutes. Some people do it while in the shower, others in the yard. You want to spit it into a trashcan, not your sink.

I can only last a few minutes while oil pulling! But I feel like it's still beneficial. I like to mix the base oil with 1 drop of clove oil or a squirt of Dentalcidin LS, an herbal mouthwash.

What's the cost?

Just the cost of the oil: $5-$20

Ozone Therapy

What is it?

Ozone therapy is the method of using ozone gas to treat medical conditions. Ozone is a colorless gas made of 3 oxygen atoms.

What's the benefit?

Ozone therapy benefits include:

- Regulating immune system
- Improving circulation
- Stimulating detox
- Increasing oxygen at cellular level
- Boosting mitochondria health

How do I do it?

Ozone therapy is an in-clinic treatment using a medical grade ozone generator. When looking into ozone therapy, be sure to find a functional medicine practitioner with ozone training or certification.

Ozone can be delivered in a variety of ways. The most popular form is autohemotherapy. This is when a patient's blood is drawn, injected with ozone, and then returned to the body. But ozone can also be delivered through localized injections, ozone saunas, ear insufflation, or nasal insufflation.

If you suffer from chronic allergies or sinus infections due to mold recovery, ozone via nasal insufflation may be particularly helpful.

What's the cost?

Ozone injections average between $30-$200, IV ozone will run anywhere from $100-$1,000 per session, and ozone sauna sessions will cost around $30-$80.

Rebounder

What is it?

A rebounder is a mini trampoline, usually used indoors.

What's the benefit?

A rebounder moves lymph and blood and helps oxygenate your tissues. It also provides exercise that helps support cellular and mitochondrial repair. It can renew your energy during your workday so you avoid using sugar or caffeine.

How do I do it?

Aim to use your rebounder 1 minute five times a day or 5 minutes three times a day. It depends on your goals if you are trying to use more for exercise, lymph therapy or just a quick pick-me-up.

If you've become exercise-intolerant due to fatigue, these little bursts of exercise give you that heart pumping, oxygen and circulation you need for detox and health without wearing you out completely. As you get healthier, you can use your rebounder as part of a HIIT (high intensity interval training) workout.

What's the cost?

$50-$150

Red Light Therapy

What is it?

Red light therapy involves exposure to low levels of red light that you can see.

Unlike the light used in tanning booths or the rays from the sun itself, red light therapy does not expose you to damaging UV rays. Instead, it directs very low levels of heat to your skin by way of a lamp, device, or laser with a red light.

What's the benefit?

Red light and near-infrared light are used to reduce inflammation, improve blood flow, heal wounds, and rebuild cells.

How do I do it?

Red light is applied through a hand-held device or a panel. There are several brand options. I use a handheld device from Sunlighten and it advises you to keep it on an area for about 90 seconds. Commercial units, like the Joov, have 15 minute sessions in which you are sandwiched between two panels.

What's the cost?

$150-$400 to purchase a unit or $30-50 at a therapy center.

Vinegar Bath

What is it?

Vinegar baths are a detox method of adding apple cider vinegar (ACV) to your bathwater.

What's the benefit?

Vinegar baths balance the body's pH, enhance immunity, soothe skin conditions, and naturally pull toxins from your body.

Your skin's pH is meant to be slightly acidic. ACV's acidity helps restore your skin's pH balance, which can ease symptoms of eczema and psoriasis and may even help prevent wrinkles.

Apple cider vinegar also has antimicrobial properties, so this bath can be especially helpful if you're coming down with a cold or virus.

How do I do it?

Fill your bathtub with hot water and add 2 cups of apple cider vinegar. If your muscles are feeling sore you can also add a sprinkle of Epsom salt to the mix.

Soak for about 20-30 minutes, or until the water becomes cool. Anne Louise Gittleman, one huge proponent of vinegar baths, recommends you not rinse off afterwards to retain the pH balancing effects. But if you can't stomach the smell, rinse off afterwards just without soap.

To enhance the bath's benefits, add a tablespoon of ACV to a glass of warm water and sip away as you soak.

What's the cost?

Just the cost of the apple cider vinegar - around $5-$10 a bottle.

SUMMARY:

You don't need to do everything on this list, but if you do a number of them I can bet you will develop your own favorites that move the needle in *your* health. You may also find other favorites not listed here.

In the next chapter, we'll tackle targeted symptoms and system repair!

Client Story –

Margo was a teen with acne, painful periods, constipation and depression. It wasn't the best way to experience her teenage years! A dedicated, daily castor oil pack routine changed all of that. She also worked on improving her diet with more real food, and took magnesium and fish oil supplements.

Simple things can make a big difference! **I recommend the organic castor oil and easy-to-use packs by Queen of Thrones.** I'll share their shop link and an interview with the founder at toxicmoldguide.com, Chapter 10, or see Bridgit's favs at bridgitdanner.com.

11
STEP 3: TARGETED SYMPTOM/SYSTEM REPAIR

IN THIS CHAPTER

- The most common symptoms of toxic mold illness: **fatigue, brain fog, weight gain, digestive complaints, chemical sensitivity, mood changes, poor sleep, hormonal imbalance, pain, altered immunity**
- Possible causes of each one
- My favorite labs, supplements and techniques for each

INTRODUCTION

THERE CAN BE some finger wagging within functional medicine that you shouldn't treat the symptom, you should treat the root cause. But the symptom is often *showing* you the root cause, or at least a short list of what could be going on.

As people tend to identify more with their worst symptoms rather than a body system malfunction, I decided to group this chapter by ten common mold symptoms. For each one, I'll discuss possible causes and solutions. In the following chapter, I'll go more into the lab testing options.

FATIGUE

Mold will affect your energy, primarily, due to lowering energy/ATP production in your cells.

This can also cause widespread systemic damage such as:

- Insulin resistance
- Low adrenal output
- Low testosterone
- Poor brain performance
- Low thyroid activity

Getting to the root of fatigue is definitely a worthy exploration and you'll likely have several factors contributing to your fatigue.

Luckily there are some things you can add to your daily routine that give you more energy through getting more oxygen or brain stimulation. And there are some general things you can do like working on your diet or utilizing adaptogenic herbs.

Beyond that it will take your long-term efforts at detoxification and your restoration of various body systems. And, for the long haul, you'll need to keep up a good diet, manage stress, move your body and get a good night's sleep.

Possible causes:

- Adrenal fatigue
- Low thyroid function
- Heavy metal toxicity

- Mitochondrial deficiency due to mold
- Leaky brain
- Blood sugar issues
- Iron deficiency (especially if out of breath easily)
- Overwork
- Poor sleep
- Chronic stress
- Cell danger response

Possible tests:

- Hair Tissue Mineral Analysis
- Blood panel, including iron, hormones, blood sugar
- Mycotoxin test
- Organic Acids test
- Non-metal toxins test (I use Great Plains; Vibrant Wellness also has an option)

Testing is covered in more detail in the next chapter.

Quick wins:

- Rebounding (jumping on a mini trampoline)
- Dry brushing
- Coffee Enemas
- Sauna
- Essential oils such as peppermint and orange
- Salt water/electrolytes
- Cold water bath/shower or cryotherapy
- Dancing
- Singing
- Morning sun exposure
- Exercise, especially right away in the morning or when you need a pick-me-up

Ideas:

- Glandular thyroid or adrenal support (I like Standard Process brand)
- Adaptogenic herbs (Siberian ginseng or maca are two ideas)
- Chlorella (detoxifies and energizes)
- Floradix, Ferrasorb (monitor ferritin levels)
- Higher fat/higher fiber diet - avoid processed foods
- CoQ10 - 200 mg day (I like our Mi CoQ10, taken first thing in AM)
- Avoid snacking - look into time-restricted eating
- Acupuncture
- My lemon greens drink (see www.toxicmoldguide.com for recipe)
- Salt, salted water or electrolytes

CELL DANGER RESPONSE (CDR)

One explanation for 'incomplete' improvements is the cell danger response (CDR), a term coined by Dr. Robert Naviaux.

Your mitochondria are the conductors of the cell danger response orchestra. When your mitochondria detect a threat, whether that be a mycotoxin or an injury, that puts the cell danger response in motion. ATP is released outside of the cell, creating an inflammatory process to shield the cell from invaders.

This means your mitochondria's ATP is redirected towards defending your cells, instead of making energy. Which is exactly why people with a triggered cell danger response feel so tired!

Common symptoms of cell danger response include:

- Fatigue
- Depression
- Brain fog
- Chronic pain
- Inflammation
- Rashes
- Digestive issues
- Autism

When the perceived threat is gone, the cell danger response can be completed. Which is why getting out of the moldy environment is the first step towards healing!

Once you are in a safe environment, you can adjust your lifestyle habits to keep the cell danger response in check. Avoiding toxins is crucial, which means a focus on eating organic, cleaning up your personal care and cleaning products, and limiting EMF exposure.

Stress can also trigger CDR, so practicing stress management techniques such as yoga, breathing, meditation, and exercise are key. Just don't overdo it though, as over-exercising can also trigger CDR. Easy does it.

Many supplements can help calm the immune response to stress, including CoQ10, quercetin, essential fatty acids, and NAD+.

BRAIN FOG

Brain fog is another common symptom. This is not a medical term, but it's become a common term describing:

- Poor recall of words, facts, or thoughts
- Feeling like you're thinking/moving through mud
- Losing things
- Can't learn as well
- Can't focus as well
- Confusion
- Can't work/think for long periods of time

Since mycotoxins can weaken and then cross the blood-brain barrier, they can cause a whole lot of trouble in the brain. Beyond issues with thinking, this can cause:

- Nausea
- Poor appetite
- Poor digestion
- Anxiety
- Muscle weakness
- Muscle tremors

Removing mycotoxins and other toxins, shoring up the blood-brain barrier, and feeding the brain the right nutrients are key.

Possible causes:

- Leaky brain (compromised blood-brain barrier)
- Head trauma
- Heavy metals or other toxins
- Mitochondrial deficiency dt mold
- Poor circulation/oxygenation
- Nutrient deficiencies
- Autoimmunities of the brain

Possible tests:

- Neuroquant
- SPECT scan
- Mycotoxin test
- Organic acids test
- Blood-brain permeability testing
- Brain autoimmunity testing

Ideas:

- High-quality fish oil - 1,000-3,000 mg/day
- Chelated magnesium or magnesium threonate - 300-600 mg/day
- Phosphatidylcholine (PC) - 1-2 servings/day (I use Pure PC by Quicksilver)
- High fiber diet (lots of fresh fruits and veggies, quinoa or buckwheat also great)
- Additional fiber from chia seed, hemp hearts or fiber supplement (I use MegaPre)
- High-quality probiotic (I like Megaspore 2/day with a protein meal)
- Higher fat/higher fiber diet - avoid processed foods and any simple sugars
- CoQ10 - 200 mg day (I like our Mi CoQ10, taken first thing in AM)
- Avoid snacking - look into time-restricted eating
- Avoid all dairy and gluten
- Focus by Human Elements (I take this daily)
- Lion's Mane & other medicinal mushrooms (see Neuro Effect by Paleovalley)
- Phosphatidylserine (PS) (See Neuro Optimizer by Jarrow)

Client Feedback on Pure PC:

"I've tried everything. The pills, shakes, detoxing, binders, sauna, ice baths, ozone, IV infusions, surgery, nasal rinsing for mold in sinuses, the list goes on & on & on. Bottom line with this product....it is doing something. My body responds immediately and I can tell it's helping."

— ELIZABETH K.

PAIN / HEADACHES

I think pain and headaches are one of the most overlooked symptoms when it comes to mold illness. Practitioners will naturally assume these are due to structural issues, stress or hormones and, occasionally, food.

While working on your physical alignment, cleaning up your diet and taking some hormone supplements may help, pain or headaches will return if you are still in a moldy environment and have Chronic Inflammatory Response Syndrome (CIRS).

I was getting multi-day headaches when I was recovering from mold illness and it drove me crazy. Recently they started up again. After some time and lots of massage, chiropractic care, heat packs and Advil, I looked more into histamine intolerance.

I realized I was getting exposed to fragrance and not eating and drinking my best. Taking some antihistamines and carefully avoiding histamine foods (see the diet chapter) did the trick 100%.

Possible causes:

- Herz reaction (side effect of too rapid detox)
- Histamine intolerance/Mast Cell Activation Syndrome (MCAS)
- Chronic Inflammatory Response Syndrome (CIRS)
- Nutrient deficiency
- Lymph congestion
- Muscle tension
- Structural misalignment
- Jaw clenching
- Blood sugar issues
- Toxin overload/ liver congestion
- Food intolerances or gastrointestinal inflammatory foods

Testing:

I don't have any specific testing suggestions; just take care of your physical health locally and follow any other testing ideas that seem appropriate for your case listed in other sections.

Ideas:

- Hot/cold packs
- Dry brushing
- Exercise (see previous chapters)
- Essential oils like peppermint or basil
- Slow your pace of detoxification

- Avoiding high histamine foods such as dairy, leftovers, salami, tea, coffee, chocolate
- Chiropractic care
- Lymphatic massage
- Acupuncture
- Physical therapy
- Cryotherapy
- Hyperbaric Oxygen therapy
- Chelated magnesium 300-600 mg/day
- Turmeric (Apex Energetics has a great liposomal version)
- Anti-inflammatory diet

Client feedback on our powdered magnesium:

> *"I have been using this product for a few weeks now and I am truly enjoying the benefits. I feel calmer, sleep better, gentle on my gut, and less muscle pain."*

DIGESTIVE COMPLAINTS

Almost everyone experiencing mold will have some digestive complaints. **Even if you don't have GI symptoms, you may still have an issue in this system, but it presents as brain fog, headaches or skin rashes.**

Digestive complaints can include:

- Loose stool
- Constipation (no bowel movement in more than 24 hours)

- Multiple food sensitivities
- Abdominal pain/discomfort
- Nausea
- Heartburn
- Poor appetite
- Weight loss or gain
- Bloating
- Brain fog
- Rashes
- Headaches/pain

Unfortunately, by the time you've discovered you have a mold problem your gut has likely become quite imbalanced. You have too much unfriendly bacteria and not enough friendly bacteria. You have a leaky gut lining and parasites. You have chronic inflammation, biofilms with mold inside, and overgrown yeast.

If that sounds awful, you're right! This is why it usually takes testing, protocols, and time to recover your gut health. Be patient as you go through this process.

It took me *years,* and gut protocols are my *least* favorite! I am very sensitive to any herbal or pharmaceutical bug killer. But now when I have consistent, formed bowel movements and my gut tests come back normal, I am so proud.

Since the digestive system is the site of nutrient absorption and production, it's important to address. The intestinal tract can be quite the source of inflammation, infection (which makes more inflammation) when it's not healthy, making you even sicker.

An increasing list of food sensitivities could be a symptom of mold illness. I had a client recently who asked if she could be cured of her food sensitivities. But most of these foods were inflammatory foods like gluten and dairy, so it wasn't so much of a sensitivity as an intolerance.

Other foods could be true allergens for you. This can be discovered through IgE blood testing. Note that there can be false positives in these tests. Eggs and nuts are common in this category.

Still more foods *do* cause sensitivities - inflammatory reactions that may not happen immediately. This can all get really confusing!

My main concern as a health practitioner is when my clients can't tolerate a long list of nutritious foods. Some clients can only tolerate three things, like broccoli, rice and chicken.

Like chemical avoidance, there may be a period of time when you have to honor these food sensitivities. **Your goal is to heal your gut and other systems enough to add to your dietary list.**

You can consider trying different diets, like the elimination diet or the low-histamine diet, and see how your body responds. Keep a food journal. You can test for food sensitivities (these can change over time) and allergies (these likely will not).

If your gut health is a constant struggle for you, I strongly recommend testing and customized protocol with a functional health practitioner. It's easy to keep spinning your wheels for *decades*, wasting a lot of money in the process.

Possible causes:

- Intestinal permeability
- Intestinal inflammation
- Candida overgrowth

- Small Intestinal bacterial overgrowth (SIBO)
- Small Intestinal fungal overgrowth (SIFO)
- H Pylori overgrowth
- Deficiency of stomach acid or digestive enzymes
- Hypothyroidism
- Food sensitivities
- Insufficient chewing
- Stress
- Celiac disease and other autoimmune digestive disorders
- Neurological issues
- Parasites and worms
- Mast Cell Activation Syndrome (MCAS)
- Loss of oral tolerance
- Dysbiosis (imbalanced bacteria)

Testing Options:

- Stool testing (we use the GI-MAP)
- Celiac and other autoimmunity testing
- Food allergy testing
- Food sensitivities
- Colonoscopy
- Endoscopy
- SPECT scan

Ideas:

- Megasporebiotic with MegaPre as directed with a protein meal (start at a lower dose)
- Biocidin tincture for infections
- Para 1-3 products by Cell Core for parasites
- Immunoglobulins such as Mega IgG 2000 (great for loose stool) & Mega Mucosa (great for inflamed gut)

- MATH diet (see Chapter 7)
- Low FODMAP diet (see Chapter 8)
- Low histamine diet (see Chapter 8)
- Chew well
- Broad-spectrum digestive enzymes (I like Digest Gold - just one per large meal)
- Supplemental hydrochloric acid (HCl)
- Prokinetics like ginger, Iberogast, and MegaGuard (can help with nausea and constipation)
- Bitters like gentian tincture
- Essential oils such as frankincense, peppermint and ginger topically (learn to use safely)
- Vitamin A - 5,000 IU/day for mucosal barrier
- Aloe vera juice
- Licorice tea
- Coffee enemas, gargling, singing and laughing (good for the vagus nerve)
- Glutathione - 100 mg/2 times a day with food
- Clean fish and fish oil - 1-3 gm/day

Client Feedback on Megasporebiotic:

"Absolutely love this probiotic. Been taking for months now. Initially I had to start slow, & gradually increase dosage (die off symptoms were heavy for me) until I could tolerate the full amount. These have helped my digestion, moods & inflammation. Definitely worth a try!"

WEIGHT GAIN/FOOD CRAVINGS/ENERGY FLUCTUATIONS

When I was at my sickest, I craved processed carbs and caffeine. I didn't go completely overboard, as I already had a firm grasp on good eating. But I needed a 'hit' of noodles at lunch and tea in the afternoon. This coupled with less exercise caused a bit of weight gain.

When your brain is starving for energy, you will crave a quick fix. **A brain poisoned by mold and struggling to do its complex processing may want sweets and treats.**

Weight gain can occur quite rapidly when in a moldy environment. Your genetics, inflammation, toxin overload, slowed metabolism and estrogen dominance can all come into play. This can make it difficult to lose weight, but as you repair various body systems, I believe it's possible.

Symptoms could include:

- Irritable if can't eat
- Craving sweets or caffeine
- Frequent urination
- Skin tags
- Weight gain focused around the abdomen
- Needs to eat frequently

Possible causes:

- Impaired detoxification
- Dysbiosis
- Increased beta-glucuronidase (this is an enzyme that can put toxins back into circulation when elevated)

- Estrogen dominance
- Decreased metabolism
- Hypothyroidism
- Insulin resistance
- Cellular energy deficit

Testing:

- Mycotoxin
- Stool testing
- Non-metal chemical testing
- Blood labs including thyroid and insulin/sugar markers
- Continuous Glucose Monitoring for 2+ months

Ideas:

- Multivitamin with chromium
- Cinnamon in tea, smoothies, tincture, capsule or food
- Castor oil packs
- Sauna
- Exercise
- Time-restricted eating
- High fiber, high fat diet - avoid processed foods and sweets
- Dry brushing, apply a bit a grapefruit oil to any cellulite
- Cold water soaks/showers or cryotherapy
- Localized cryotherapy treatment
- Lymphatic massage
- Digestive enzymes with meals
- Brush teeth after meals
- Chew xylitol gum and drink water between meals
- Brisk walk after meals
- Essential oils like grapefruit, lemon, or peppermint to combat cravings

- Berberine before carbohydrate-rich meals (not for daily, long-term use)

Feedback on our Hi-Potency Multivitamin:

"Fantastic - by far the best multivitamin I've ever tried. That, in addition to the megaspore, have catapulted my midlife weight loss efforts into a new zone. Thank you Bridgit and team ☺"

— AMANDA S.

Continuous Glucose Monitor (CGM)

Recently I have been using a CGM with the goal of stabilizing my blood sugar to heal my brain/energy issues. A CGM is a wearable device that adheres to the backside of your upper arm. It has a tiny, flexible needle and some circuitry that collects data, in the case my blood sugar levels, that uploads to an app on my phone. I bought mine for a 3 month period from an online site called NutriSense.

I have learned *so* much from wearing my CGM. I have learned:

- Carbs are better processed in the AM than the PM
- I'm sensitive to fruit, white rice, potato, processed flour, sugar and alcohol

- I need way more protein than I thought
- A big, rich multi-faceted meal can work well for me
- Snacks may be good for me, as long as they aren't carbohydrate snacks

Using a CGM isn't about counting calories and doesn't have to be about losing weight. It's about learning what meals prevent or encourage an inflammatory spike of high blood sugar. These spikes are not good for brain health and can lead to insulin resistance.

I honestly feel everyone should use a CGM for a few months...but only if you are motivated to actually make changes. If you are reading this book, you probably are!

I assumed I was doing a lot of things right with my diet, but I was off the mark in some ways. I think many 'healthy' people will notice the same. Purchasing a CGM is a great way to know for sure and prevent the metabolic issues that plague us modern humans at an alarming rate.

IMMUNE/RESPIRATORY ISSUES

Your immune system will take a serious hit from chronic mold exposure, as we covered in Chapter 3. This is yet another pattern where the root cause of mold will likely not be found by the conventional medical system. Patterns of:

- Asthma
- Stuffy or runny nose
- Frequent colds and flus
- Frequent mucus
- Frequent clearing of the throat
- Chronic sore throat
- Airborne allergies

May actually be due to mold/mold illness.

These symptoms could also be caused by other airborne irritants like pollution, smoke and fragrance.

Testing:

- Mycotoxins
- Non-metal toxins
- OAT test
- MARCoNS
- Blood testing - WBC panel, vitamin D
- Food sensitivity testing
- Food allergy testing
- Epstein Barr virus

Ideas:

- ACS Silver nasal spray by Results RNA
- Silver mouth throat spray
- Herbal throat spray (I like Megacidin and Biocidin throat sprays)
- NeilMed nasal irrigation (similar to a Neti pot)
- Mouth taping
- Astragalus (I like Mediherb brand)
- Antioxidants - glutathione, zinc, vitamin A, E, C, D (I like 5,000 IU/day of vitamin D when not in summer sun)
- Nettles
- Quercetin
- Avoid dairy products and sugar

As I mentioned in my story, I had some asthma symptoms return after twenty years a few years back. Airborne mold, chemicals, pollen and other irritants can trigger asthma. There is also something called leaky lung (increased lung vascular permeability) that can come into play.

Earlier this spring I took a cocktail of antioxidants for leaky lung, which somewhat helped. I also have two inhalers, which I would like to ultimately no longer need.

Next allergy season I plan to take more of a histamine management approach and see how that goes. Balancing hormones, perhaps with supplemental progesterone, can also help us midlife women who have an increased chance of developing allergies and asthma thanks to estrogen dominance.

Client feedback on ACS Silver Nasal Spray:

> *"I got this product to see if it would help with a chronic nasal infection. The infection was one of those that didn't block my breathing, but left me always clearing my throat of the post-nasal blobs. I tried the Neilmed irrigation, which helped, but didn't kick it out. With ACS Spray (and still using Neilmed) - the white blobs are almost completely gone. YEA. No more having the clear my throat all the time!"*

Client feedback on Biocidin Throat Spray:

> *"I was very impressed with how fast this spray works. I felt a cold coming on and after using this in less than 24 hours felt I had it under control. I would recommend this spray to everyone."*

MENTAL HEALTH ISSUES

With the stress of a moldy home and body, you are likely to experience overwhelm, anxiety and depression. I endeavor to help you with that throughout this book. However you can also approach these issues with herbs and other natural remedies.

Beyond a 'manageable' level of mental health challenge, you can develop crippling symptoms or even fully diagnosable mental health conditions such as schizophrenia.

I remember admitting to my husband that I was so exhausted that I fantasized about never having to wake up. I had these vague ideas of how to do it. Head in the oven? Bottle of pills? I wasn't really going to do it at that point, but it scared me enough that I thought I should tell him.

When I told him, instead of freaking out, he admitted that he saw things that weren't there. We both were experiencing mental health challenges. This could manifest as:

- Suicidal ideation
- Anxiety
- Depression
- Insomnia
- Depersonalization/dissociation
- ADD/ADHD

- Bipolar disorder
- Weepiness
- Anger

Testing:

- Neuroquant
- SPECT scan
- Environmental toxins tests
- Blood-brain permeability
- Autoimmunities of the brain
- Psychiatric evaluation

Ideas:

- Avoid alcohol and processed foods, especially food additives of any kind
- Meditation
- Heartmath
- Apollo Neuro device
- Guided visualization
- Therapy
- Coaching
- Melatonin (can even be taken in daytime for anxiety)
- GABA
- L-theanine
- St. John's Wort (do not mix with antidepressants)
- Phosphatidylcholine (Pure PC 1-2 servings a day)
- Detox, detox, detox! Sauna, castor oil packs, dry brushing, binders, clean diet...all of it.

If you are experiencing mental health challenges, it's critically important you get out of a moldy environment now. If your child is experiencing behavioral changes, you need to move out.

Children's brains are still developing - being chronically exposed to a neurotoxin at this time can lead to permanent brain changes. Remember our lessons in part one of this book; find something temporary as you look for a longer-term housing option.

I am not a mental health professional and I highly encourage you to find one you like if you or a family member is experiencing new mental health symptoms. The therapy I received about a year into mold illness was really helpful and I regret not starting sooner.

The national suicide hotline number is 800-273-8255.

CHEMICAL SENSITIVITIES

If you weren't already, you may find that now you are super sensitive to scents and chemicals.

This could look like:

- Headaches
- Anxiety
- Racing heart
- Nausea
- Feeling faint

Or other symptoms.

This likely will happen right away when you encounter the chemical, but it could also be delayed. This is sometimes referred to as Multiple Chemical Sensitivity (MCS).

Multiple chemical sensitivity is not an allergy. Instead, people with MSC have neurological reactions to environmental toxins - whether that be pesticides, fragrances, or toxic mold.

With all the chemicals in our modern environment, Multiple Chemical Sensitivity has shot up by 300% in just the past decade! In fact, just under 26% of Americans report they are chemically sensitive.

Huffing chemicals certainly isn't good for any of us! **We should all avoid using toxic cleaning products and using perfumed, highly-synthetic beauty products.** If you need help with cleaning up your routine, stay tuned; in two chapters I'll cover it.

But a sensitivity can get really hard to deal with when you can't stand to be around a swimming pool or can't visit a hotel.

While you are at your sickest, avoidance may be needed at whatever level is needed for you. You simply cannot be in an environment that's going to get you sicker.

After mold exposure, your body sees foreign, airborne material as a threat, and it may overreact. It's releasing inflammatory factors and perhaps adrenaline. Over time, as you detox and heal, hopefully these triggers will get at least tolerable. For some bodies, letting go of this overreaction is challenging.

There is some body of work that helps retrain your response to these triggers. Annie Hopper founded the Dynamic Neural Retraining System (DNRS), a healing approach to rewire patterns in the brain as seen in Chemical Sensitivities. My friend Dr. Eva Detko offers a program as well to train the energy body after chronic illness and trauma. These courses are both online.

There is also biofeedback and Eye Movement Desensitization and Reprocessing (EMDR).

Explore the options that appeal to you. I included some links in the online resource section. I find that investing in my self-awareness and emotional healing is always worthwhile!

Testing:

- Non-metal environmental toxins test with organic acids test (Envirotox)
- Neuorquant

Ideas:

- Open windows
- Use an essential oil diffuser or an air purifier in hotel rooms
- Limit time in questionable environments
- Meditate
- Change HVAC filters every 3 months and choose a high rating of purification for your filter
- Wet mop and wet dust regularly or have a cleaning company do so
- Be cautious with materials if remodeling or building a home (more in Part 3)
- Use a HEPA vacuum at home
- Avoid all toxic and scented products
- Repair your gut
- Therapy for any past traumas
- Limbic system retraining program

POOR SLEEP

Sleep is a super important time for your healing. I find many clients resist taking anything to help them sleep, thinking it's addictive or unnatural. Don't do this! If you can't sleep, take action.

Ever since my life got more 'adult' I've had trouble on and off with sleeping. Now I know that something is off with my situation or mindset if I'm not sleeping well. At other times, I'm on the brink of my period or I had too much caffeine or sugar, so I can't sleep.

Your reasons for poor sleep can vary and bounce around. I take sleep aids as needed, and even carry them with me when I travel. I take baths at night, read and meditate. But if I still need a little something to help me sleep deeply, I have zero regrets about using these aids. Getting my beauty sleep is keeping me perky and glowing at 47.

Causes:

- Worry/rumination
- Stress/high cortisol levels
- Low melatonin production
- Parasites
- Inflammation/pain
- Digestive upset
- Circadian rhythm disruption

Testing:

- GI Map stool test
- DUTCH hormone test (includes cortisol and melatonin)
- Sleep study for sleep apnea

Ideas:

- Melatonin 3 mg* (I like Melatonin-SR by Pure Encapsulations)
- Epsom salt baths
- Essential oils of lavender or sandalwood
- Chelated magnesium 300-600 mg/day
- High magnesium foods such as spinach, almonds and pumpkin seeds
- Avoiding sugar, alcohol and carbs in the evening
- Avoiding caffeine completely or after noon
- Trade coffee for green tea (more calming)
- ½ t nutmeg in warm nut milk with honey before bed
- Adaptogenic herbs like ashwagandha (I like Sleep Maintenance by Gaia Herbs)
- Qualia Sleep supplement
- Get enough physical activity in the daytime, but not at nighttime
- Not over exercising (inducing keyed-up, healing state at night)
- Sauna in the evening
- Mouth taping
- Sex

*I find that many people are wary of supplemental melatonin. Fear not! Melatonin is produced less with age and you may be producing even less if you have nasal or gut infections related to mold. Melatonin is a super beneficial antioxidant with many functions in the body, including immune support. Low levels of melatonin, along with vitamin D, are associated with COVID severity.

Still can't sleep?

You may need some OTC sleep or allergy medication on some nights. Don't get in the habit, but do it if you need it. I have a few clients on Rx sleep aids. I don't think these are usually needed but if your case is extreme, like you are getting 0-3 hours a night, talk to your doctor.

HORMONAL IMBALANCE

Some common symptoms:

- Low libido
- Loss of muscle
- Infertility
- PMS
- Irregular periods
- Difficult menopause
- Man boobs
- Delayed or early puberty
- Acne
- Excess hair growth or balding

As you learned in Chapter 3, hormones can very much be disrupted by toxic mold. Toxic mold, along with other toxins, are underappreciated causes of the rampant weight gain, infertility and erectile dysfunction in our modern culture.

Of course, hormonal issues can also be caused by poor diet and stress, and aging will play a role as well.

We produce hormones at all ages and stages of life, so levels will vary depending on your age, and even the types of hormones produced will change. Keeping my hormone levels up as I age has been really helpful in feeling youthful, energetic and athletic.

Testing is incredibly helpful in addressing hormonal imbalance. Having reviewed many test results with clients, what we experience in symptoms does not always match the test results. You can get some critically important information with testing!

For me, stress and toxicity have made my hormones low, low, low for years. I was working as a hormone and fertility specialist, and I felt that taking bioidentical hormones was 'giving up' or 'cheating.' But when I finally tried them for about 6 months, it was game changing.

I now know it's important to keep an open mind about treatment options. **Don't let your own judgements about how medicine 'should be' limit your recovery.**

Testing:

- Blood labs (see next chapter)
- DUTCH urinary hormone test

Ideas:

- Essential oils such as clary sage for PMS and peppermint for hot flashes
- Maca Harmony (menopause)
- Broccoli sprout and seed 1-3 day (estrogen and chemical detox)
- Resveratrol (excess estrogen)
- Hemp seeds and hemp oil

- Borage oil
- Avoid dairy, sugar and alcohol (super helpful for acne and perimenopause)
- Choose wild or organic - for meat and dairy especially
- Avoid all synthetic fragrance and mainstream beauty products
- Avoid snacking and practice time-restricted eating
- Exercise
- Dry brush
- Sauna
- Castor oil packs
- Coffee enema
- High fat, high fiber diet
- Meditate
- Hormone replacement therapy
- Libido-Stim F or M by Designs for Health (herbs plus DHEA)
- Acupuncture

CONCLUSION

- We each have our own worst symptoms and most affected systems
- It will take some time to plug away at healing various body systems
- Everyone's best solutions will be different
- Take your time to try various things and find your best route

---

In the next chapter, I'll go deeper into some of the lab options I mentioned in this chapter.

I know the many suggestions above may seem overwhelming. Take a light attitude and just try one thing at a time. Or you can book a consultation with us to get our custom suggestions. We offer a few ways you can work with us through the 'lab testing' section of our shop at bridgitdanner.com.

Client Story –

William felt better after moving out of a moldy apartment, but he still didn't have the energy he wanted for working out, playing with his kids or even sex. He also still felt a bit off at work, had food sensitivities and used the bathroom too many times a day.

Testing revealed that his hormone production was low and testosterone was getting converted to estrogen. He also had several gut infections. He worked with us, as well as a local, functional physician, to boost his hormone levels and repair his gut.

William is feeling pretty much 'normal' now and he maintains a healthy routine of exercise, sauna, whole foods, supplements and an early bedtime.

12
MORE ABOUT LAB OPTIONS

IN THIS CHAPTER

- Details on testing options and companies
- Information on interpreting some lab markers

INTRODUCTION

IN CHAPTER 2, I covered testing for mold and mycotoxins in detail. But you'll likely want to test other body systems as well.

As I've explained, the body can't necessarily just right itself as you detox; it's going to need specific support in removing infections and replenishing hormonal and nutrient deficiencies.

The following are tests that I run or have some knowledge about. This is definitely not a comprehensive list! For example, there are many more options with stool testing and food sensitivity testing. Some of these options may be great; I just don't know them all.

BLOOD TESTS

Blood testing provides an accurate snapshot of your current levels of various things. You can find systems that are struggling and nutrient deficiencies.

Below are some tests I run or that other practitioners commonly run. Nowadays, in many states, you can order your own tests online. If you feel you know how to respond to the results, self testing may be a great option for you.

A lab we use is Ulta Labs, but there are others too. If you have an HSA payment card with your insurance, you may be able to use it for your own labs, health coaching or supplements.

We currently offer a couple of pre-loaded testing packages at our site which makes it easy and you get a consultation with us to review the results and make a plan. You can also ask your physician to consider some of the tests below:

- Full thyroid panel with thyroid antibodies (see below)
- White blood cell count (WBC) with differentials (gives a sense of overall immunity and possible infections or imbalances)
- Vitamin D (I like levels at 60-80 ng/mL)
- Ferritin (iron stores - 30-80 ng/mL depending on who you ask! Ferritin combined with a full RBC panel is an important check for energy in mold illness)
- HA1c, fasting glucose, insulin (also super important, especially with aging, fatigue, & weight)
- Testosterone, DHEA, estrogen, cortisol (your MD could run for you)
- Epstein Barr viral panel (this is a common, active co-infection with mold)

- Lyme-related infections (Vibrant Wellness, Igenix or Armin Labs)
- Autoimmunity testing - can identify multiple predictive autoimmune antibodies up to 10 years before onset of illness (Cyrex)
- Blood-brain barrier testing - assesses breach on blood-brain barrier due to stress, trauma, and environmental toxins and risk of neurodegenerative diseases (Vibrant Wellness or Cyrex)
- Food allergies and sensitivities (Vibrant, Cyrex and the MRT from Oxford Biomedical)

These are the thyroid labs I like to run and the ranges I like to see:

Reverse T3	>10:1 ratio to Free T3 or 9.21-24.1 ng/dL
T3 Total	100- 180 ng/ dL
Free T3	>3.2 pg/mL
T4 Total	6-12 mcg/ dL
Free T4	>1.1 ng/dL
TG AB	<= 1 iu/ml or below range
TPO AB	< 9 iu/ml or below range
TSH	1-2 miU/L

*Please note the units of measurement may be different in other countries or with other labs.

Sometimes you think it's your thyroid and it's not!

We created a lab package called Thyroid Plus for our clients that also covers ferritin, blood sugar, vitamin D and more. Thank goodness we did, because it can be disappointing to expect to see thyroid woes and see nothing.

Fatigue, weight gain, brain fog, menstrual issues - these *can* be thyroid issues, but they can also be thanks to toxicity, poor gut health and blood sugar issues. Like it or not, sometimes it takes a handful of tests to get to the bottom of things.

URINE TESTS

Dried Urine Test for Comprehensive Hormones (DUTCH)

Our favorite hormone test is the DUTCH test, which stands for Dried Urine Test for Comprehensive Hormones. This is a convenient, at-home test that covers a variety of hormones and their metabolites in a very sophisticated way.

This is currently our top-selling test at our website, which goes to show how much our hormones are driving us crazy!

The DUTCH hormone test is a complete, one-day hormone test that includes:

- Estrogen (neither men nor women want too much!)
- Estrogen metabolites (how you break down and detoxify estrogen)
- Testosterone (both men and women need to have enough)
- Progesterone (important for fertility and in perimenopause)
- DHEA (a sex hormone precursor)
- Cortisol (needed for energy, sometimes excess in stress)

- Melatonin (an antioxidant that helps you sleep and more)
- Some vitamin & neurotransmitter markers
- and more.

Organic Acids Test

The organic acids test (OAT) measures the presence of 76 metabolic markers in your urine to give an overall snapshot of your health. Organic acids, also known as metabolites, are by-products of your body's metabolism.

The organic acids test can uncover missing pieces of your health puzzle, including factors that impair detox pathways. The OAT test offers helpful insights about:

- Intestinal yeast and bacteria overgrowth
- Glutathione levels
- Nutritional markers
- Antioxidant deficiencies
- Neurotransmitter levels
- Krebs cycle dysfunction
- Fatty acid metabolism
- Oxalate levels (correlated with chronic illness)
- And much more!

GPL-Tox Test - Toxic Non-metal Chemicals

Every day you're exposed to hundreds of toxic chemicals. They're in our food, water, household products, pharmaceuticals, personal care products, and even the air we breathe! These toxins slowly accumulate in your body and wreak havoc to many bodily processes - especially detoxification.

Getting a clear picture of your own body's toxic load can serve as a helpful baseline, making treatment more effective and gentle. That's where the GPL-Tox test comes in. This test uses 18 metabolites to screen for 173 different environmental toxins - all from a single urine sample.

The GPL-Tox test will uncover levels of:

- Organophosphate pesticides
- Phthalates (found in most personal care products)
- Benzene (product of car exhaust and industrial processing)
- Xylene (found in paint, pesticides, cleaning products, perfumes, and much more)
- Pyrethroid insecticides (found in bug spray, bug bombs, and flea/tick products)
- Vinyl chloride (used in the synthesis of commercial chemicals)
- Styrene (found in plastic manufacturing and building materials)
- Acrylamide (found in plastics, food packaging, nail polish, and cosmetics)
- Tiglylglycine (a marker for mitochondrial disorders)
- And much more!

Heavy Metals 24-Hour Urine Test

Heavy metals are found in food, water, chemicals, environmental pollution, paint, medicines, dental care, cosmetics, and much more. When your body accumulates too many heavy metals it can have disastrous effects on your health, causing neurological symptoms, chronic inflammation, inability to detox, digestive issues, muscle pain, and fatigue.

If you suspect harmful heavy metals could be part of your health puzzle, Great Plains Laboratory offers a 24-hour urine test that checks your levels of:

- Mercury
- Lead
- Cadmium
- Arsenic
- Chromium
- Copper

These heavy metals build up over time and hide in your body's deep tissues.

For that reason, this test is best used with a metal detoxification agent such as DMSA or EDTA. These sequester the hidden metals from your deep tissue and mobilize them to be excreted in your urine.

Collection is timed over a 24-hour period to allow the most accurate results possible.

HAIR TESTING

Hair Tissue Mineral Analysis (Helpful for Mineral Balancing & Heavy Metals)

Another great option for checking heavy metals is to do a hair tissue mineral analysis, known as HTMA. Your hair is one of the places your body eliminates minerals and heavy metals. For that reason, the HTMA can reveal both heavy metal toxicity and mineral deficiencies.

An HTMA test can also provide helpful information about:

- Metabolic rate
- State of stress
- Energy levels

It's important to choose a company that doesn't wash the hair at the lab, as this affects the test's accuracy. For that reason, two labs I trust for HTMA are Analytical Research Labs (ARL) and Trace Elements (TEI).

STOOL TESTS

GI-Map Test

Your gut health impacts your digestion, neurotransmitter levels, hormone production, energy levels, blood sugar, immune system, inflammation, nutrient absorption, and much more.

So obviously, if something is impairing your gut health, you want to know! There are several stool tests on the market. Some are more consumer-based and focus on dietary recommendations.

We currently use the GI-Map test as it's a strong tool for a practitioner looking to help 'rebuild' a client's gut and address any pathogens.

Diagnostic Solutions Laboratory offers the GI-Map and they use a unique qPCR technology that analyzes DNA to uncover exactly which pathogens are present in your sample, and in what amounts.

The GI-Map Test looks for a wide variety of pathogens including:

- Protozoan parasites
- Parasitic worms
- Clostridium difficile
- H. Pylori
- Candida albicans
- Microsporidium

Plus, this test gives insights into:

- Bacterial health of the large intestine
- Pancreatic enzyme production
- Fat digestion
- Gut inflammation
- GI immune system health
- Beta-glucuronidase (a marker of estrogen & phase 2 liver detox)

There's even an add-in option to test zonulin, which gives helpful clues about your gut permeability. If you suspect a leaky gut is part of your health challenges, I highly recommend getting your zonulin checked.

SCANS

SPECT (Single-Photon Emission Computed Tomography)

SPECT is a powerful brain mapping tool that evaluates the blood flow and activity of the brain. This state-of-the-art test shows which areas of the brain work well, which are working too hard, and which are not working hard enough.

SPECT is used to evaluate changes in the brain due to Alzheimer's, head trauma, stroke, seizures, Lyme disease, brain inflammation, chemical exposure, and yes...mold toxicity! SPECT offers valuable information about brain health, but the downside is it's pricey. An average SPECT scan ranges between $1,300-$3,500.

If you're interested in getting a SPECT test done, my recommendation would be Amen Clinics.

Neuroquant MRI

Neuroquant is a software that measures brain volume from a specific type of MRI scan. Mold illness affects the permeability of the blood-brain barrier, which can cause structural changes to the brain. If your mold illness manifests with cognitive symptoms like memory issues, confusion, and word recall this test can help.Neuroquant data can be analyzed to determine the severity of mycotoxin effects on the brain.

According to our colleague, Dr. Mary Ackerly, a Neuroquant MRI can be fairly affordable around $300.

Client Stories –

We have many satisfied clients who have run tests with us! Here are a few quotes from our website:

DUTCH:

" I am so happy with my Dutch test consult with Micki, she was so helpful in her explanations and was easy to understand. This is my 2nd Dutch test and I love to see the progress and changes that I made in one year. Thank you Micki, I am looking forward to trying your suggestions and hopefully will resolve my sleep issues. Gratefully, Colleen"

GI-MAP:

"The (GI-MAP) test was quick, easy, and had results pretty fast. So many things showed up! Micki helped me interpret the results and make a plan to get my stomach straightened out. Currently

on week 4 of the protocol, and there is already a HUGE difference. My digestion has taken a full turnaround and I'm able to live normally without thinking of bathroom visits. So grateful for this test and Micki's help!!" • Kelci

MYCOTOX TEST:

"Working with Bridgit was great! She was really knowledgeable and committed to providing detailed, actionable information. Even better for someone like me who has been to several doctors before, she showed a lot of empathy, interest and genuine concern in really digging into my history, symptoms and test results to come up with the best plan possible." • Julie

THYROID PLUS TEST:

"This was a very complete test and included so much more than just thyroid. The results came directly to me by email and were very clear and easy to read. Of great value was the half hour thorough analysis session with Bridgit Danner. She was very engaging and was able to make many suggestions. I found her very friendly and focused. I had her complete attention and it was most refreshing. I even received follow-up notes after the time she had already given me." • Marlo

PART III
DEVELOP

I know it may be hard to believe when you're in the thick of the mold mess, but your life will get better. It will calm down and get more normal. But it will never be quite the same.

Every event changes us. Mold may change your physical resilience for the worse, but your mental resilience for the better. It may have taught you to cook and sunbathe, and removed a few of your 'friends.' It may have cost you thousands of dollars, but you gained a new outlook on life.

These last few chapters are about *your* next chapter.

They are about:

- Avoiding other toxics that will strain your body
- Learning how to heal when you're still wobbly
- Creating your best life with intention and discernment

You may be tempted to skip these chapters! I encourage you to curl up with a cup of tea and finish them out when the time is right.

This trauma you lived through is not meant to be just survived; it's meant to make you superhuman.

13
AVOID ALL TOXINS

IN THIS CHAPTER

- Identify toxins to avoid in your home
- Identify workplace toxins
- Water filter options
- Ingredients to avoid
- EMF considerations

INTRODUCTION

IF YOU HAVE BEEN AFFECTED by toxic mold, you know how powerfully damaging toxins can be.

In your own home, as a mold sufferer, it's important to become aware of all possible sources of toxicity, both natural and manmade. These intermingle in a toxic soup of triggers to your struggling immune system.

Here are just a few stats to paint a picture of the toxin overload we face today:

- The EPA chemical inventory lists 84,000 potential toxins you may encounter every day.
- There's an average of 700 synthetic chemicals in the human body.
- The Environmental Working Group states that the average woman puts 168 chemicals on her body every day.
- In 2020 alone, 68 million TONS of pollution were emitted into the atmosphere by the US alone!

The EPA and other bodies may say that the low doses are not harmful. But the trouble often lies in the combination of many, many low dose exposures, and that's hard to measure with formal studies.

According to Dr. Joseph Pizzorno, author of *TheToxin Solution*, toxins have become a primary driver of disease. Toxins' harmful effects on health have been brought to light in recent years - especially in the courtroom.

In 2015, the World Health Organization recognized glyphosate, the most commonly used pesticide, as a likely carcinogen. Soon after, makers of Roundup, the glyphosate-based weedkiller, faced claims from 125,000 Roundup users that believe the product caused their non-Hodgkin lymphoma. In several cases, judges ruled in favor of users, awarding them up to $25 million in punitive damages for their pain and suffering.

Glyphosate doesn't just increase your risk of cancer; it also kills your beneficial bacteria. Studies have connected its use with a host of health problems, including depression, mitochondrial dysfunction, hormonal imbalance, infertility, impaired liver function, and autoimmunity.

BPA is another common toxin we encounter, most often in plastic food containers and canned goods. BPA is a hormone disruptor that has a structure similar to estrogen. It binds to estrogen receptors, impacting growth, reproduction, energy levels, and much more. BPA is also considered an obesogen linked with obesity.

None of this is meant to scare you. Just give you the facts so you can make decisions. While we live in a toxic world, our daily choices have a *huge* impact.

In fact, one study found that people that avoided packaged products for just three days had decreased BPA in urine by 66%! Lesson: your actions DO have the power to transform your health.

Detoxification supplements and techniques are great and should be a lifelong habit, but toxin *avoidance* is the most efficient way to detoxify!

SOURCES OF TOXINS

You can be exposed to toxins anywhere. I'll cover some sources outside of your home, but I'll primarily focus on helping you lower your toxic load within your home for the rest of this chapter.

Workplace

Your workplace's toxic load depends on the space and the activities going on there.

Did you know being a homemaker can be one of the most toxic jobs? That's because there can be so many 'home pollutants.'

Any building can be a source of toxins thanks to water damage, the off gassing of chemical-ladened carpets, cabinets, poor air circulation, inadequate cleaning, toxic cleaning supplies, etc. In 1986, the World Health Organization coined the term 'sick building syndrome' to describe the phenomenon of people getting sick as a result of buildings.

Any building is at risk, from warehouses to schools to office buildings.

Here is a partial list of jobs with toxin exposure:

- Homemakers
- Stained glass and glass manufacturing positions
- Jewelry manufacturing positions
- Drivers
- Mechanics
- Flight; pilots, airport personnel, flight attendants
- Aestheticians
- Nail technicians
- Agricultural workers
- Office workers (sick building)

If you work in a profession that has an increased exposure to toxins, consider your current state of health and if the exposure is manageable for you at this time.

Do you need to take a leave of absence, or find a new career? Or manage your existing exposure and do more daily detox?

These decisions are very case-by-case, but, as I discussed in earlier chapters, your health is the most important factor.

Outdoors

Indoor air quality is now worse than outdoor air quality by concentration of contaminants, but outdoor air quality is still very much of a problem that does not get enough media coverage.

The results of toxins testing we do on our clients is troubling. We commonly see additives to jet fuel and gasoline in our clients' results. This doesn't seem to correlate with living near a highway or airport; it just happens.

I live in Phoenix, Arizona, a nice, dry area in regards to mold. But Phoenix is a valley that collects a lot of pollution. And it's also an environment with a surprisingly large amount of pollen.

As I write this, it's monsoon season, and a recent storm trapped more ozone in the air, which seemed to really irritate my newly re-developed asthma. I have to avoid the outdoors altogether occasionally.

When I studied COVID-19 when it first emerged, I learned about the correlation between particulate matter in the air and increased infection in an area. It concerns me how this particulate matter can burden our lungs and immune systems, and it can especially affect children, the elderly, low-income and the chronically ill.

Action items:

- How is the air quality in your area? Have you looked up any statistics?
- Does outdoor air quality ever seem to bother you or your kids?

- Do you ever stay in when the air quality index is poor, or use a mask outdoors?
- Is it time to see an allergist or a pulmonologist?
- Do you need to apply the respiratory health tips in the chapter on targeted treatment?

Indoors

This is our area of concentration, as we spend on average 90% of our time indoors, and most of our time at home.

I find that people often skip ahead to the question of, 'which air filter should I buy?' but this is actually my last consideration.

First you need to evaluate all sources of indoor contamination, and then minimize them. Since we've been covering air quality, let's continue with that subject within your home.

Air

As we covered in Chapter 1, a toxic mold colony does not just bring mycotoxins, but VOCs (volatile organic compounds), spore fragments, bacterial endotoxins, etc.

Within your home's air there could also be:

- Dust
- Dust mites
- VOCs from furniture and fabrics
- Skin scales
- Pet dander
- Yeasts
- Chemicals
- Allergens
- Artificial fragrance
- Pollen grains

Meanwhile those gasoline fumes and particulate matter from outside are getting inside, too. You can imagine it's all a lot for your system to process!

To keep down indoor airborne trouble makers, consider:

- Repair sources of water damage
- Optimize air circulation and humidity
- Perform frequent cleaning, including wet mopping and dusting, with non-toxic products
- Reduce synthetic materials in the home (example: choose cotton or wool area rugs over synthetic)
- Choose less toxic building materials (example: ceramic tile instead of laminate)
- Choose less toxic furniture (example: choosing real wood over particle board)
- Change air filters (every 3 months) and clean air ducts (every 2 years)
- Use a higher quality air filter rated MERV 11 or higher
- Open windows and doors
- Run a HEPA filter
- Move if your building is an issue
- Replace old mattresses and use a dust cover on mattresses
- Wash linens regularly
- Wash seasonal clothes before wearing again
- Do not use artificial air fresheners, candles or scents

Many contaminants will settle in the dust in your home, so it's important to wet dust, wet mop and HEPA vacuum frequently. If you don't love to clean, consider an outside cleaning service.

I have a great little crew who come twice a month, happily use my non-toxic cleaning products, and clean things I would never get to, such as my ceiling fans and window shutters. It's worth every penny!

Educating on the above topics gets quite in-depth, so I like to bring in outside experts. If you haven't tuned into my Toxic Mold Masterclass, you can access some of these expert interviews at the book resources page.

Water

"Which water filter should I buy?" is a common client question. It's a great question, but the answer is not super simple.

How you obtain filtered water depends on your water source, your budget, and if you rent or own your home.

Two resources to investigate your water are:

- Your municipality's water report (search online for your community report)
- My TapScore (private testing company)

If you use well water, you'll need to test yearly and maintain your treatment system. Local testing is likely available in your area, or you can use www.mytapscore.com.

As with well water, treating city water should ideally match your water's conditions. This involves testing and then a customized solution. But this can be expensive.

Issues with city water can include:

- Pesticides & herbicides
- Pharmaceutical residue
- Heavy metals
- Water treatment chemicals (chlorine, chloramine)
- Fluoride
- VOCs

Your municipal water report will not include all these elements. Options for filtration include:

- Whole house filter
- Sink reverse osmosis
- Bottled 5 gallon jugs
- Pitcher filters (carbon filters)
- Showerhead filters
- Bottled spring water

It's important to remember that you absorb and breathe in water while bathing - it's not just drinking water that's the issue.

So if you are not investing in a whole house filter, please use a showerhead or bath spout filter for bathing. (One brand for this is Aquasana.)

So far in my lifetime I have used:

- Brita filters (these don't do much)
- Purchased filtered water in refillable jugs
- Berkey filter
- Whole house filter with sink RO (reverse osmosis)

- Whole house filter with no sink system

I also used some kind of Peace Corps issued filter in South America...but that's a different story.

In my last home, we had a whole house filter and a sink reverse osmosis. It was great in theory, but it was expensive to install and changing the filters was a whole plumbing situation that I don't want to ever deal with again.

Currently I have a whole house filter made by iSpring that I purchased from Home Depot online. My fridge is on a kitchen island, so installing a reverse osmosis that would 'feed' the ice maker and water dispenser would be tricky. So I skipped this and opted for a whole house filter that seemed good and back-washes itself. I don't need to do anything with the filter for 10 years!

Ideally, I would have tested my water and retested again after installation. And I know my carbon filter is not removing some things in my local water, like arsenic. But it's still a nice filter that solves at least some of my problems, it was in my budget and is easy to maintain.

These are some of the decisions you need to make along the detox journey. You probably can't afford every amenity and that's ok. Just do your best and let yourself off the hook for the rest.

INSPECTING YOUR HOME FOR TOXINS

Food Supply Tips

It's not just what you eat, but what your food is touching and how it's processed.

- Avoid take-out containers and 'heat-up' containers - this 'paper' is coated in toxins
- Bring your own travel mug to the coffee shop (this got shut down during COVID)
- Eat in
- Swap out all the plastic kitchen items that you can for glass or metal
- Avoid the microwave
- Avoid processed foods and food additives
- Eat organic, wild, grass fed and local
- Avoid conventional non-stick pans
- Store dry goods in glass containers

Medicine Cabinet Ideas

Learn non-synthetic alternatives to avoid the dyes, fillers and side effects from OTC medication.

- Nasal rinse or silver nasal spray
- Reusable heat packs and ice packs
- Essential oils like peppermint for headaches and stomach aches and lavender for bug bites
- High dose fish oil and magnesium for inflammation and pain
- Quercetin for allergies

Three essential oil authors I like are: Dr. Mariza Snyder, Jodi Cohen, Dr. Eric Zielinski.

Cleaning Products Ideas

Some good, synthetic fragrance-free brands are:

- Branch Basics

- Seventh Generation
- Aspen Clean
- Better Life
- Biokleen

Be a cautious consumer; many brands want to capitalize on the 'green trend' but they are not 100% green. A 'tell' I look for is added fragrance. If a brand has some harmful ingredients withheld, but still adds synthetic fragrance to its formula, I call BS and put it back on the shelf.

Ingredients to avoid:

- Formaldehyde
- Ammonia (ammonium hydroxide)
- Fragrance ("parfum" or "scent")
- Chlorine bleach (sodium hypochlorite)
- 2-Butoxyethanol (ethylene glycol monobutyl ether)
- Triclosan
- Ethanolamines
- 1,4-Dioxane

You can also make your own cleaning products with white vinegar, baking soda and essential oils.

Better Beauty Products

Finding natural beauty products that perform is a favorite hobby of mine! There are more and more great brands with true ethics around sustainability as well as products that really work. Allow yourself some trial and error as you find your new favorites.

Brands I like:

- Beautycounter
- Eminence
- Young Beauty
- Annmarie skincare
- Giovanni hair products
- Weleda
- Dr. Bronner's
- Just Nutritive
- Everyone soaps & lotions
- Just the Goods
- Be Green Bath & Body

Ingredients to avoid:

- Fragrance or parfum (these are always synthetic and contain phthalates)
- Parabens
- Phthalates
- Oxybenzone
- Formaldehyde
- Ethanolamines
- PFAs and PFCs
- 1,4-Dioxane
- Butylated hydroxytoluene (BHT) and butylated hydroxyanisole (BHA)
- Carbon black
- Siloxanes
- PEG compounds
- Sodium lauryl sulfate

When in doubt, look the product up on the EWG's "Skin Deep" database to check the safety rating at ewg.org/skindeep.

Garage

Garages can contain some of the most toxic products! A few you may need, but, again, there are often less toxic alternatives.

Weed Killer:

- Mulch regularly to avoid weeds
- Cover low lying weeds with newspaper (the lack of sun will kill them)
- Soak weeds with vinegar
- Clove oil - add 10 drops to a spray bottle, fill with water, shake well & spray away
- Roll up your sleeves, break a sweat, and dig them out!

Insecticide:

- Diatomaceous earth
- Neem oil
- DIY Soap spray - Add 1 tbsp Dr. Bronner's soap to a quart-sized spray bottle and fill with water.

EMF

Electromagnetic fields, or EMFs for short, are invisible fields of energy created anywhere electricity is present.

Power lines, cell phones, microwaves, televisions, computers, and all other electronics emit these invisible streams of energy. The closer these electronics are to your body, the more EMF exposure you face.

While these gadgets are handy and part of modern life, growing research suggests EMFs are bad news for your health. Studies have linked EMF exposure with an increased risk of cancer and neurological problems like depression.

Everyone is exposed to EMFs daily. But it hits some people harder than others. People sensitive to EMFs may show symptoms such as:

- Insomnia
- Headache
- Depression
- Fatigue
- Difficulty concentrating
- Memory problems
- Dizziness
- Irritability
- Restlessness or anxiety
- Nausea
- Skin burning or tingling

You may have noticed a lot of those symptoms are similar to mold toxicity! Speaking of mold, research has found EMFs can amplify mold growth, causing it to spread more rapidly.

EMFs can also hit people with a leaky brain especially hard. This is because research shows that EMFs increase the permeability of the blood brain barrier.

While you can't avoid EMF exposure altogether, there are a number of things you can do to reduce it:

- Put your phone on airplane mode when you're not using it
- Turn off your Wi-Fi router at night

- Use the speaker function or earbuds when chatting on the phone
- Don't carry your phone in your pocket - put it in a purse, bag, or briefcase
- Invest in a radiation-blocking cell phone case like
- Don't sleep with your phone in your bedroom
- Unplug regularly - do a digital detox when you can

If you are extra sensitive to EMFs you can even consider hard wiring your internet, rather than using Wi-Fi.

CONCLUSION

Let your home be as safe of a haven from chemicals as is possible. This helps your body recover, avoid symptom flare-ups and helps prevent degenerative diseases down the road.

- You can't completely avoid toxins, so make detox habits lifelong - sauna, green drinks, etc.
- You don't have to update every aspect of your home at once; just do what you can step by step
- Little changes add up to more and more toxin avoidance!

Client Story –

Feeling run-down, Marta started researching online for answers. She knew her diet could be better, so she joined a meal planning service. She was surprised to find so much information about toxins in everyday products, and she swapped out her cleaning and beauty supplies with fervor.

Her husband groaned when she wanted to hardwire the internet, but he was content with TV and cell phone in the end. Still, she was experiencing thinning hair, increasing weight and deep fatigue.

When she found out about mold, a lightbulb went off. She lived in Florida, where humidity was constant, and their home had been through more than one storm. When they did find mold, it was stressful, but her husband, a contractor, took on the project.

They moved to a nearby town they had their eyes on anyway, and they are both happy. Marta's hair is growing back, and the couple spends more time riding bikes and visiting the beach than they had in years.

14
STAGE OF HEALING

IN THIS CHAPTER

- The benefits of a daily routine
- How to do more things, little by little
- Balancing realistic and ambitious goals
- How to handle set-backs
- How to create metabolic resilience

INTRODUCTION

HEALING your body will be a roller coaster, but you can make it a kiddie roller coaster and not that great big loopy-do roller coaster by practicing awareness and good habits.

You will have good days and bad days. You will get frustrated and sad. But you will also spend a full day at the lake with friends and not get tired, or concentrate on a project for hours without even realizing it.

Have you ever seen the bikes they have for kids called balance bikes? They have no chain or pedals, the kid just glides or pushes. It's a much more effective way to learn to balance on a bike, and it's less stressful than dealing with the pedals.

This is you. Your body is your bike. You are learning to glide and balance, but for now you need to help yourself out a bit because you're still wobbly.

STAGES OF HEALING

It's hard to say which symptoms or systems will get better for you first - I think it's very case-dependent. I've read that some systems will be in a different stage of healing than others; for instance, your gut health could be improving at a much faster rate than your endocrine (hormonal) system.

Roughly, there are these 3 stages:

1. **Severe:** this is when symptoms are at their worst, with many symptoms, debilitating symptoms, and/or lack of ability to function (this could be body systems or your ability to work, move, etc.)
2. **In Recovery:** this is when you have regained some function and see improvements, but you aren't where you want to be and can have flare-ups from triggers like work, exercise or scents.
3. **Maintenance:** In this stage you are mostly better, but likely you still have to guard your health in various ways. There could be some symptoms and triggers, but the list is shorter and less severe.

Notice I did not put any time frames on these stages, as lengths of time will vary.

The most important way to move out of the severe stage is to get out of a moldy environment.

Also not mentioned was the pre-discovery stage. If you are *lucky*, you will notice symptoms and consider your building within a few weeks or months.

But most people are not in that scenario and spend years in a dangerous environment. It's usually not until symptoms are severe that mold may come up as a possibility, and even then you could spend years without considering mold.

HEALTH IS NEVER STATIC

The state of your health is *always* changing. You may wish to go back to your early 20s when you could stay up late partying and still wake up early and put in a full day's work!

First of all, I sincerely applaud you for wanting that energy back. Many people accept ill health and low energy as a normal part of aging, and it's not.

Although you can't go back to that age and state, you can have really high energy again, but you won't get there with late nights of partying.

Other events will affect your health too - injuries, childbirth, a move to a new climate. **Rather than long for the past, focus on your current health goals.**

Here's another example from my own story. I'm nearly 5 years out of a moldy home, and my health is pretty darn good. But some things that do bother me, nearly every workday, are severe energy dips and brain fatigue. I will hit the wall with a tension headache and a complete inability to do any more mental work around 4 PM.

Honestly I'm not sure how much of this has to do with mold, but it doesn't really matter. My health goal is to have more sustained energy in the day, and kick the headaches.

I have tried hyperbaric oxygen (I literally bought a tank for my house) and it wasn't a big help. I did get some useful tips in physical therapy and currently am doing some big diet experiments with low-carb eating, ketosis and fasting that seem to help.

So I keep 'goaling' and exploring all the time. I'm not *constantly* doing a big experiment; I pursue new goals organically, like I taught you. But I never give up on feeling my best, and I make new discoveries and have wins all the time.

ROUTINE VS. VARIETY

When you are at your sickest, or even as you go about your workday, sticking to a routine is best. When you honor natural circadian rhythms for sleeping, eating and working out, it creates less stress for your body and you can heal more quickly and experience less side effects.

This is the equivalent of gently patting along the ground as you balance your bike, in the simile I shared above.

You can build up to having more resilience by practicing something called hormesis.

> "Hormesis refers to adaptive responses of biological systems to moderate environmental or self-imposed challenges through which the system improves its functionality and/or tolerance to more severe challenges."
>
> — MATTSON MP. HORMESIS DEFINED. *AGEING RES REV.* 2008 JAN;7(1):1-7. DOI: 10.1016/J.ARR.2007.08.007. EPUB 2007 DEC 5. PMID: 18162444; PMCID: PMC2248601.

Hormesis can be practiced with some things previously mentioned like sauna, cryotherapy, fasting and breathing exercises.

We humans also need variety. Going to a new restaurant, away on vacation, or dancing the night away makes life more interesting.

As your health gets stronger, you can try more of these things. Per our balance bike example, this is picking up your feet and enjoying some glide time!

I would suggest not trying too much at once. For example, if it's your first time eating out in a while, at least stick to a healthy menu item, so no fries, milkshakes or even soy sauce. If you stay out late, be home by 10 PM instead of 1 AM.

Trying new things may make you feel worse. It's a bummer, but really it's just information. You are not quite ready for that activity, at least for now.

If you are experiencing a set-back, feel the feeling, but don't make a big story about it.

Have a little cry, get it out, and then take a walk, pet your cat or make a cup of tea. Enjoy what you can on a bad day. Know that you'll find answers later.

Don't beat yourself up that you can be 'just like everyone else' and do whatever you want all the time. First of all that's a fantasy, and second of all treating your body carelessly will likely send you into early aging and chronic disease.

Be proud of how far you've come, and also of your healthy moderation.

There may be some things that you will always have to be careful about. For me, I have to watch my travel habits. Late nights, early mornings, cold airports, restaurant food and too much social time throws me off hard. I do my best to fly in the daytime, bring warm clothes, sleep in and take my supplements!

CONCLUSIONS

- Mold is not your only health factor
- Know that the road to healing is bumpy and that's normal
- Find your personal balance of routine vs. variety
- Healing from toxic mold illness takes time
- Don't beat yourself up for not being like 'everyone else'
- There is no such thing as perfect health
- You are in a long-term relationship with your own health. Show up for it.

My Recovery Story

At first I had a very gradual improvement in energy and brain function. My eyelid also stopped twitching. And I stopped having the suicidal thoughts that came from extreme fatigue.

I was out of my house by then; we were in a temporary house that was a lot better but we brought too many moldy belongings there, which was a mistake. We were there for about 5 months.

I think my next big turning point was when we took a 2-month road trip. The new environment helped, and the fresh air. I joined a Pilates studio for a month, and I got stronger and stronger, and lost a few pounds. I moved from 'severe' to 'recovering.'

But I also still had a sore throat and post-nasal drip and I got my first urinary tract infection ever, which required 2 rounds of antibiotics. My immune system was weak.

When we got back to the Pacific NW, I was able to work but I had high anxiety, headaches, and still had sore throats. It was a bit of a backtrack to be in a wet, cold, stressful environment.

Moving to Arizona later helped somewhat. My main symptoms were cleared enough that I noticed all the other nagging symptoms. **This was one of the hardest periods because I was out of the trauma of mold, but not as healthy as I hoped.** I suppose you could call my first couple of years in Arizona 'late recovery stage.'

One symptom I took forever to find answers about was headaches. I had strings of them and it took *all these years later* to get that it was a histamine problem. And I'm a practitioner. Lately I'm taking a daily Claritin and not getting recurrent frequent pseudo-flus either.

It took me *years* to find mouth taping for my chronic sore throats. But now I don't have them at all. It's the best thing ever. And I'm so thankful I keep learning so that I keep feeling better.

15
CREATING A NEW LIFE YOU LOVE

IN THIS CHAPTER

- Assessing what's working and what's not
- Identifying limiting beliefs
- Trusting that answers will come
- Following your spark of interest
- Being open to BIG changes

INTRODUCTION

IN THE THROES of your darkest days of tossing out mementos, wondering where you'll live, and if your brain will ever work again, it may be hard to believe that your new life will be better than what came before.

But for me, and many of my clients and friends, our lives *are* better than ever! I once heard Tony Robbins say that your future is always better than your past because you've grown. That new version of you will naturally call in better things!

Don't neglect your growth. Growing involves feeling painful feelings and making uncomfortable choices. It's not exactly fun, but it's expansive.

REFLECT ON YOUR LIFE

We often move from one day to the next, or one thought to the next, without much reflection.

A chronic illness, big move, divorce, job loss or other life stressor is an opportunity to look at what you believe and what is, or is not, serving you.

You may love your life, and feel cheated it's being 'taken away from you' by mold. Or you may be happy that mold gave you a chance to make a welcome exit!

Consider these five areas:

Mindset

This is firmly the #1 most important thing to consider, but also the most elusive. Your thoughts are so automatic, your beliefs so deeply ingrained, that they seem to be 'you.'

They are not you. They are habits and learnings. They are changeable - if you review them and decide to do so.

Here are some considerations:

- Do you expect yourself to be perfect?
- Do you keep your word even when it's costing you?

- Do you drive yourself relentlessly and ignore your need to rest?
- Do you allow time for chats with strangers and laughs with your kids?
- Do you spend time judging or gossiping?
- Do you compare yourself to others and always fall short?
- Do you have a negative body image?
- Do you worry about things you can't control?

What thoughts do you want to have?

I'm thinking of a couple of friends whose kids are younger than mine. They are great moms and rooted in that identity. They host perfect holidays and have their kids in all the sports.

They are holding it all together with an iron grip, and this is the blind spot. This tight control of creating a perfect life removes time for rest, spontaneity, romance, health and friendship - or at least some of those things.

I know how that goes because I was once that overworked supermom. Some years and one divorce later, I see quite clearly the risk of neglecting other areas of your life.

Now let's say that supermom is going through mold (I was her once too). She may try to control her way out of it and re-establish that perfect life for her kids. But her health and relationships are probably suffering like never before, and questioning her mindset and her priorities is a fantastic idea!

Of course she should invest in her kids while they are young, and she may need to sacrifice some 'me time' in this stage of life. But here are a few changes supermom could make:

- Establishing a bedtime routine of baths, reading, and meditation instead of ice cream and Facebook (bedtime routines aren't just for kids!)
- Scheduling a babysitter and asking her hubby to plan a date night
- Asking for help when she needs it
- Saying no to connections that don't serve her
- Having a fixed monthly girls' brunch
- Prioritizing some daily outdoor movement
- Getting outside help with cleaning and food preparation
- Hiring a life coach
- Not taking the small details of life too seriously
- Enjoying music, dancing and play time
- Reviewing and planning her week to ensure she prioritizes herself

The above is just an example - I don't mean to pick on moms.

Single people (I'm in that category now), may be out of the house a lot, traveling, drinking and eating at restaurants. Or they may fall into habits of eating alone in front of the TV and not socializing.

And *all* of us can hang out in negative self-talk and a fearful avoidance of change.

If this kind of self reflection is new to you, I applaud you for getting started! Taking even a little time to assess how you show up in life, and if it's working for you, is powerful.

Health Habits

Obviously you will need to review your health habits when faced with mold. But health maintenance is a forever thing, and I think it's important to have a holistic, self-supportive system in place for the long haul.

Like I mentioned in the exercise section, your needs depend on your personality. You might need external motivation and support, or prefer solitary activity.

- How were your habits before mold?
- What habits do you want to keep going years from now?
- What are your current and long-term health goals?
- Do you eat for emotional reasons?
- Do you snack out of boredom?
- Do you know how to cook?
- Have you found a workout you enjoy?
- Do you prefer group exercise, therapy or meditation?
- Do you love having a personal trainer or a massage therapist?
- What blocks your healthy habits?
- If you fall off track, how quickly do you get back on?
- How well do you follow a healthy routine on an average day?
- Do you drink due to social anxiety, or have a heavy-drinking social group?

One of your biggest 'mold wins' can be carrying forward new healthy habits for life.

Physical Surroundings

This includes your home, state and country. This is a great time to question your attachment to home and location and what it's really about.

Questions:

- **If you could live anywhere, where would it be?**
- What sentimental value does your home hold?
- Is your home cluttered?
- What financial loss or gain would you take if you moved, if any?
- Do you fear loss of friendships and community if you move?
- Are you afraid of getting out there and forming new friendships?
- Do you truly love the community and neighborhood you live in?
- Are you ready for a change?
- Is there another state or country you're curious about?
- Is it time to downsize?
- Is it time to go completely nomadic?
- Would you prefer to live with other family members, like your daughter or aging parents?
- Would you rather be in the country or city?
- Would you like access to bike paths, public transit or hiking trails?
- Would you like more time in the mountains or at the beach?
- Would you like to be a house sitter or to live in a guest house?
- Could you do an academic residency or sabbatical?
- What 'stuff' really matters to you, and what doesn't?

I realize that right now you may be literally homeless or staying on someone's couch. Imagining a ski town lifestyle may seem out of reach. But I invite you to enjoy that imaginative process.

What aspects of it light you up? If you can't have the ski chalet immediately, can you take a walk in a forest this weekend and smell the pines? Connect with what brings you joy and keep moving towards that bring you more joy.

Once you open up to your desires and creativity, you may be able to manifest something better than you ever thought possible!

Career

You will likely spend many years of your life working, so you want that work to be meaningful to you. It doesn't matter if it's meaningful to anyone else - just you.

Many of us study or start out in one career only to realize it's not the right fit. And something that's a fit for 10-20 years could stop being a fit, too.

Now is a great time to ask if you're satisfied in your career, and if it supports your health.

When your whole world is upended by mold, consider:

- What do you like or not like at your current job?
- What tasks do you most like to do?
- Do you prefer company or working alone?
- What would you most like to do?
- How do you want to spend your days?
- Do you like to be moving or still?
- Would you prefer a couple of part-time jobs or just one?

- How many work hours are ideal?
- What kind of schedule would you like to have?
- Are you interested in training for a trade or specialized job?
- Do you want to freelance or start your own business?
- Would you like a different position at your current company?
- What are your natural talents and acquired skills?
- How could you make the most use of your time for money?

Again, I appreciate that right now you may not be able to work at all. It sucks. But you will be able to work again, so you get your creative juices flowing and start researching and manifesting!

People

There is a lot of talk on social media about removing toxic people from your life. But the first person to look at is you. No one is perfect; we all have our unhealthy reactions and attitudes.

Before you go blaming everyone for being toxic, realize that everyone is just human. Every adult is a grown-up, wounded child.

I used to be the queen of taking everything personally. It caused a lot of stress. Now I'm much better at seeing that when someone is being rude, it's likely that they are triggered or having a bad day, or I'm triggered or having a bad day, or both!

Every experience is filtered through your own lens. When you can blur the lens a bit, it takes that painful, sharp-edged experience of life away. Everything is in the grey, not black or white.

Especially now, in our ultra-divided society, it's great to learn to appreciate various perspectives. You don't have to change your view, but just allowing others to be, without harsh judgement, is better for your nervous system and health.

It's not about approving of things you don't respect, it's more about respecting yourself enough to not waste your precious energy getting all riled up.

So I'll frame the questions below about how you want to be, as well as who you want to be with:

- Do you take things personally?
- Do you often judge others throughout the day?
- Are you a good listener?
- Do you show up for your friends and family?
- Do you try to fix others who didn't ask for it?
- Do you do community service work?
- Do you have at least one close friend you can confide in?
- Do you make an effort to meet new people?
- Do you focus on where life is lacking?
- Do you give thanks for your blessings?
- Does your spouse or significant other support you?
- Are you walking on eggshells for anyone in your life?
- Is anyone putting you down or starving you of love?
- Do your friends or family talk about you behind your back?
- Are the people in your life petty or uplifting?
- Do your friends talk about big ideas or do they gossip?
- Do you have friends you can have adventures with?

- Do you spend time with people you don't like just because you have a history with them?
- What kind of friends would you like to have?

Just like junk food will drain you, being around the wrong people will drain you too. You may have some friends who are nice enough, but you've just outgrown them. That's ok.

You usually don't even have to say anything to slowly spend less time with them. You can simply decline some invitations, and start making plans with new groups or friends.

You only have one life to live - find your best people!

You may be dealing with some really toxic 'mold doubters.' Don't waste energy on them if you can avoid it. Your job is not to convince anyone. Just take care of yourself and keep it moving!

OUT WITH THE OLD, IN WITH THE NEW

In order to usher in something new, we need to get rid of something old. Again, what we hold dear is often automatically decided based on beliefs developed in childhood. Here were some of mine:

- I can't leave my patients
- I can't sell my clinic
- I need a partner to be whole
- I can't take criticism
- People don't respect me
- Everyone leaves me

When I write these down, it's embarrassing! But it's an important first step to identify your limiting beliefs. Our beliefs are so ingrained that we don't even *know* them, never mind question them. If it starts with 'I can't,' odds are it's a limiting belief.

I hear these with clients about all sorts of things:

- I can't move now
- I can't leave this job
- I can't move my kids
- I can't stop eating bread and cheese
- I can't get rid of my sewing collection

As a coach, it's tough to get through this brick wall of belief!

Try This Exercise---

There's an author named Byron Katie who has an exercise called 'the work' to help you question your thoughts.

First you identify the thought, then ask yourself:

1. Is it true?
2. Can you absolutely know that it's true?
3. How do you react when you believe that thought?
4. Who would you be without the thought?

> Spoiler alert: none of it is true!
> Impossible things can become possible
> when you question your beliefs.

Here's another spoiler: avoiding that hard thing that needs to be done will not make it go away. You can delay it, and suffer in the meantime, but it won't go away.

If you find yourself overthinking and justifying and not doing what you know is in your best interest, recognize that. These hard, right decisions are always rewarded. Maybe not right away, but they are.

Here are some examples of changes people have made:

- Let go of toxic people and found better people
- Moved to a new state and made a new beginning
- Built an amazing home from scratch
- Switched to a more fulfilling career
- Became a self-care expert
- Became a more easygoing and peaceful person
- Prioritized nature and outdoor adventures
- Prioritized time with family and friends
- Started volunteering
- Became a guide for other mold sufferers
- Became a health care provider
- Gained an uncluttered, low-tox home
- Got pregnant
- Enjoyed a nomadic lifestyle

Here's one example of a big win in my own story:

Some years back, a friend of mine, Dr. Mariza Synder, recommended a daily journal called *Speed Dial the Universe*. Mariza is an amazing manifestor who turned a troubled childhood and overworked early adulthood into a very fulfilling life.

I used this journal everyday while I was trying to sell my wellness center in Portland. Mind you, I'd tried to sell it before, unsuccessfully. I'd already dealt with tire-kickers and withering interest.

The clinic wasn't super profitable, but it was busy, and clients and staff were happy, so I didn't want to close it in order to move to the drier climate of Arizona.

Everyday I wrote out my vision of selling the business, along with my daily to-do list and gratitude list. Again I got tire-kickers. Meanwhile I was working hard and was anxious about mold illness and my marriage. But I persisted.

Eventually, I meant a tenacious New Yorker who expressed sincere interest. But I was not an easy audience; I had heard it all before.

Her trip to come visit got waylaid, but she insisted she would buy my clinic, sight unseen. We signed an agreement online, and she drove across the country in her Prius and wrote me a check. She now owned the clinic and I drove away in a moving van towards Arizona *that same day*.

My clinic became her new start, and the sale provided me a new start with my online business in a new state.

The clinic is still serving its neighborhood, and I'm super happy about my Arizona life and my online business, which allows me time for rewarding projects like this book.

YOUR TURN

If you got this far, THANK YOU for reading. I feel honored to share with you and serve you.

Your mold journey may drag on a while until you find your happy ending. **But I truly believe you can make lemonade out of your moldy bowl of lemons, and I'm cheering you on 100%.**

YOUR TURN

I would LOVE to hear about your wins. You can share with me @bridgit_danner on Instagram or in our Facebook 'Mold Recovery Group.' In the event that these links change, we will keep you updated at the online resource center for this book, www.toxicmoldguide.com.

I have a large collection of blogs at bridgitdanner.com where you can research specific topics. I'd love to have you keep learning with me by joining my newsletter at bridgitdanner.com or toxicmoldguide.com.

As I keep learning, I keep sharing. And I love learning from you as well; I am constantly inspired by the dedication and creativity of our clients and community members.

Bridgit Danner, LAc, FDNP

ACKNOWLEDGMENTS

My clients & online community

Travis & Lincoln Danner

John & Karen Beasley

Dr. Mariza Synder

Alex Dunks

Tami Wilson

Mindy Palmer

Dylan Howard

Taylor Kilmer

Melissa Cardenas

Maelyn Villanueva

Micki Contini

Dr. Peter Kan

Dr. Jay Davidson

Dr. Datis Kharrazian

Dr. Ritchie Shoemaker

Dave Asprey

Dr. Susanne Bennett

Dr. Neil Nathan

Dr. Robert Naviaux

Michael Rubino

Matt Pratt-Hyatt

Dr. William Shaw

JW Biava

Kirin Krishnan

Bethany Lucas

Amanda Baldwin

Dr. Margaret Christensen

Dr. Gail Clayton

Dr. Anna Cabeca

Brian Karr

Celeste Fine

Bill Baren

Evan Brand

Ari Whitten

Connie Zack

Rachel Fresco

Kelly Kan

Joyce Steindler

Lara Adler

Jeffrey May

Jason Prall

Joe Rignola

JJ Virgin

Sai Leigh

Linsi Brownson

Jennifer Eaton

And anyone else I missed…thank you!

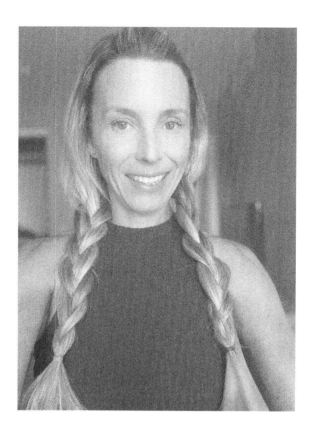

ABOUT THE AUTHOR

Bridgit Danner was working as an acupuncturist when she discovered toxic mold in her 100-yr old home and began the long journey of home and body repair.

Bridgit loves to teach about everyday detox, functional living, and toxic mold illness. She is also the founder of a line of mold detox supplements called Functional Detox Products.

She lives in Arizona with her son, two dogs, and a Soronan desert tortoise.

:|: Instagram: @bridgit_danner :|: Website: bridgitdanner.com :|:

Made in the USA
Las Vegas, NV
24 August 2023

76571781R00184